Low Carb
Lifestyle
&
Weight Loss
Made Simple

Zane Griggs

Disclaimer

This book contains the ideas and opinions of its author based on his personal experience and study. It is not intended to replace the advice of the reader's physician or medical professional. Please consult your healthcare provider before following the advice in this book and if you have any specific health conditions or concerns. The author and publisher specifically disclaim any responsibility or liability for injury or loss incurred as a consequence, either directly or indirectly, by the reader in the use and application of the advice in this book.

Cover Photo: Shannon Fontaine
Cover Concept: Danielle Griggs

Low Carb Lifestyle & Weight Loss Made Simple by Zane Griggs

ISBN 978-0-578-46915-7
© 2019 Zane Griggs. All rights reserved.
Second Edition
Published by Zane Griggs
www.zanegriggs.com
✉ zane@zanegriggs.com
facebook.com/zanesblog
youtube.com/c/ZaneGriggs
instagram.com/zanegriggsfitness

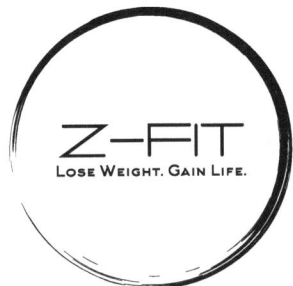

*This book is dedicated to my wife, Danielle,
for her energetic patience and grit.*

*And to my kids Amanda, Zachary, Isabella and Jett.
You inspire me.*

Acknowledgments

I would like to thank Stacy Brickell for the brainstorming sessions for this book as well as the daily planner that goes with it, despite her being a busy mom of 4 and working on her Ph.D. Thank you Bob Heilig for encouraging me to get out of my comfort zone because playing small doesn't serve anyone. To my buddy, Chance Scoggins, thank you for the encouragement, straight talk, swift kicks and saying "your first book".

CONTENTS

Foreword.. vii

Introduction.. 1

Chapter 1 The Skinny on Low Fat Diets........................ 5

Chapter 2 Low Calorie: How Low Can You Go?........... 11

Chapter 3 We Are Not Alone...................................... 16

Chapter 4 High Fat, Low Carb..................................... 21

Chapter 5 Obesity Is a Form of Internal Starvation..... 27

Chapter 6 Intermittent Fasting................................... 31

Chapter 7 What About Exercise?................................ 36

Chapter 8 When Is the Best Time to Eat Carbs........... 46

Chapter 9 Sleep Tight... 49

Chapter 10 How Do Know How Much Fat or Carbohydrate I'm Eating?.. 52

Chapter 11 Let's Go Shopping..................................... 56

Chapter 12 The Meal Plan... 61

Chapter 13 Let's Eat. 68

Chapter 14 Time to Get Moving.................................. 81

Chapter 15 Put the Plan and the Planner to Work 83

Recommended Books... 87

References... 88

Daily Planner.. 90

Foreword

One of the greatest travesties in modern health is the last 35 years of nutritional science that we have been given from mainstream media and pop culture.

Prior to the 1950s, really before mass agriculture hit scale, the obesity rate for adults in America was less than 5%. Today, rates are approaching 1/3 of all Americans.

Diabetes rates are at all-time highs and no disease will outpace diabetes worldwide over the next 20 years. A planet filled with chronically elevated blood sugars is fueling the flames of chronic disease and mortality.

But why?

How have we become fatter than we've ever been in the history of mankind, while simultaneously eating less fat than in all of documented human history?

How, in a world where there are multiple billion dollar pharmaceutical companies that treat diabetes, heart attacks and strokes, is there continuing to be a rise in all of these diseases?

With so much noise around the topics of fitness and nutrition, it's not hard to understand why most people are confused.

Here's the truth: all calories are not created equal, and if your primary weight-loss strategy isn't to fix your diet first, you will not win.

This book will eliminate the confusion and quiet all the noise for you. Zane has a mastery of nutrition and how it affects your fitness goals. He's also made it very simple to follow the rules with his play-by-play plan.

— Aaron Wenzel, MD
Board certified Family Medicine
Founder/CEO Brentwood MD

INTRODUCTION

You can't go back and make a new start, but you can start right now and make a brand new ending.
                                                    -James R. Sherman

Are all of the conflicting messages about a healthy lifestyle, weight loss and the correct way to eat just confusing you and causing you to wonder if anyone really knows how our bodies work?

Do you feel like you've tried every diet, occasionally with some moderate success but ultimately the weight still comes back?

Does it seem like no matter whose advice you follow, nothing seems to work for you?

Let me begin by apologizing on behalf of the fitness and weight loss industry for the mixed messages and false advertising about how we should be eating for both weight loss and general health. The frustration and anxiety you may be feeling is normal and unsurprising.

I began working as a personal trainer in 1998. The majority of my clients wanted to lose weight. The problem was, at the time, I had no clue about how we're supposed to eat to get our bodies to burn fat instead of storing fat. My understanding was that giving specific advice about diet would be outside the scope of practice. Personal trainers are not required to learn an extensive amount about nutrition or how to eat in order to lose weight.

Unfortunately, most of the concepts on which nutrition is taught and the majority of the messages you read and hear from the medical industry and government health organizations are based on studies which were completed five decades ago, some of which were misinterpreted or misrepresented. Current research, as well as research from the last several decades, would show these popular concepts to be false.

This situation is beginning to change. In an opinion piece for the Vancouver Sun Dr. David Harper states "In Canada, there are presently more than 2,600 physicians and allied health professionals who are using ketogenic (low carb) diets to reverse disease."[1]

My first experience with the benefits of a low carb diet for weight loss was in 2002. My wife, Danielle, had given birth to our third child and was struggling to lose the pregnancy weight. She was working out and eating a "balanced diet" like she had before but for some reason the weight wasn't coming off. The Atkins Diet© had become popular again a few years before this so she decided to try it and the weight came off. When I mentioned this to some of the other trainers I worked with they looked at me like I was crazy and some even said the diet was dangerous. The problem was, it worked.

I was fortunate to have the opportunity to work with participants on seasons 1 and 4 of the popular weight loss show, *Extreme Weight Loss*. I learned a lot and I'm very grateful for that experience. There was, however, a divide between what Chris Powell, the host of the show, and I knew would work and the official nutritional guidelines. Following the official guidelines, the nutritionist assigned to the show recommended a "healthy" breakfast of orange juice, toast and egg whites. This was for a 500lb man with the goal of losing half of his bodyweight in a year. *Really?* Needless to say, that wasn't what Chris or I recommended.

My frustration with the ineffectiveness of the standard dietary recommendations motivated me to dig deeper and look for more progressive sources of information about how our bodies respond to food. Food is information and what we eat sends messages telling our bodies whether to store or burn energy. The food we eat can also affect which diseases we get, how long we live and the quality of our lives. I don't think I'm alone in my belief that many of the diseases associated with aging are a result of our food choices.

I believe it is important to understand how our bodies work in order to make good choices about what we eat. When you understand how your body works, you're in a better position to determine if a particular food plan (diet) is going to be effective. You will also be able to make better decisions about what you eat in situations that are out of your normal routine. This knowledge is empowering! No matter where you are, even at a dinner party or a restaurant, you are in control. It is not difficult to understand, and once you do, you will be able to take greater control of your health.

The food plan outlined in this book is not for everyone. If you are a 19-year-old college athlete, a fitness competitor or training for a triathlon you will have different energy needs and performance goals than a typical adult who may or may not exercise and is primarily concerned with maintaining a healthy lifestyle and controlling bodyweight.

Once we understand that obesity is a hormonal imbalance, we can begin to treat it. If we believe that excess calories cause obesity, then the treatment is to reduce calories. But this method has been a complete failure. However, if too much insulin causes obesity, then it becomes clear we need to lower insulin levels.

-Jason Fung, M.D., Author

There are two very popular approaches to diet that I definitely do not recommend and which I explain in chapters 2 and 3.

However, I have found that a low or controlled carb diet to be very effective for the majority of people I have worked with who wanted to lose body fat and maintain a healthy, active lifestyle. This is NOT a short-term diet. I have eaten this way for many years because it gives me more control over my body composition and more consistent energy throughout the day compared to when I consumed a higher carbohydrate diet.

The most important concept which I hope to communicate in this book is that weight control is not a battle of calories. It is a battle of hormones. These hormones are greatly affected by what we eat as well as other lifestyle factors like sleep, stress and exercise. This is why true weight loss and weight control must be a lifestyle change and not a short term diet that is left behind as soon as the weight loss goal is hit or the frustration with maintaining it becomes too much. When you decide to change your lifestyle, you not only lose weight but you also gain control of your health.

The food we eat goes beyond its macronutrients of carbohydrates, fat and protein. It's information. It interacts with and instructs our genome with every mouthful, changing genetic expression.

-David Perlmutter, M.D., Neurologist, Author

CHAPTER 1

THE SKINNY ON LOW FAT DIETS

Character cannot be developed in ease and quiet. Only through experience of trial and suffering can the soul be strengthened, ambition inspired, and success achieved.

-Hellen Keller

The primary idea behind the low fat diet concept is that *a calorie is a calorie*. According to this belief, it doesn't matter what type of food you're eating, all calories are the same. If you eat more calories you will gain weight and if you eat fewer calories you will lose weight. A gram of fat provides about nine calories of energy. A gram of carbohydrate and a gram of protein each provide about four calories. Since fat has more calories per gram, the idea is that limiting the amount of fat we eat will decrease the amount of calories we take in and allow us to lose weight.

This is an extremely oversimplified view of how our bodies work. In fact, it is so simple that it is completely false. Are we supposed to believe that 300 calories of broccoli will affect our bodies the same as 300 calories of a fat free candy? Our bodies are not closed systems, like machines, which treat all forms of energy essentially the same way. I promise not to get too *sciencey* on you but this is important to understand. We have hormones, which react differently depending on what is going on in our bodies at that time and what we are consuming for fuel.

When it comes to fat storage or fat burning, insulin is the hormone which makes the greatest impact.

When we eat sugary or starchy carbohydrates, insulin is released to move this quickly digested energy out of our bloodstream and into muscle cells, the liver and fat cells for storage. Too much sugar is toxic to our systems and if we didn't store it shortly after eating, we would have too much floating through our bodies. Generally, the sugar or starch we have eaten is more fuel than we can use at that particular moment so any release of fat from our fat cells, and therefore fat burning, is impaired until insulin levels go back down.

Sugar and starch have the greatest effect on insulin. Protein causes a much smaller release of insulin and fat causes little to no release of insulin when eaten. So if you ate a spoonful of fat, like butter or coconut oil, insulin wouldn't be spiked, the fat you just ate would remain in your system to be used for energy AND your body's release of fat from fat stores would also continue.

You can see why a calorie is definitely NOT a calorie. The type of food you eat can determine whether you are storing fat or releasing it. If the majority of your diet is made up of a nutrient that inhibits fat burning, can you see how that would keep you from losing weight and could actually cause more weight gain?

But Weight, There's More......

Over time, our bodies don't respond to insulin as well as they did when we were younger. This is especially true if we over consume sugars and starches on a regular basis. Our muscle cells and eventually our fat cells become immune, or resistant, to the insulin transporting the energy to those cells. This is called insulin resistance. Insulin resistance can eventually lead to Type

2 Diabetes. You can have some degree of insulin resistance and never get diabetes but you will likely be carrying some extra fat weight.

Our pancreas responds to insulin resistance by secreting even more insulin to get the muscle cells to respond which works temporarily but the cycle of insulin resistance continues. The result is that the amount of insulin in our system continues to increase.

A very simplified version of the pathway to fat storage caused by insulin resistance looks like this. Insulin transports the glucose from the bloodstream to the liver and to muscles all over the body to refuel them so we will have readily available energy to move. Insulin resistance keeps the muscle cells from responding and receiving the glucose so insulin takes the glucose to the fat cells where it is stored as triglycerides (fat). Insulin resistance can also occur in the liver causing more metabolic issues. If you are carrying more than 20 lbs. of excess fat you may have some degree of insulin resistance.

This low-fat idea that's been drummed into our heads and bellies is completely off-base and deeply responsible for most of our modern ills.
-David Perlmutter, M.D., Neurologist, Author

The rollercoaster of blood sugar and insulin often causes inconsistent energy levels and frequent hunger. Many people find that a couple of hours after eating a starchy breakfast they are hungry again and wanting a snack before lunch which starts the process all over again.

So why have we been told to follow a low fat diet for the last 40 years? The crowning of the low fat diet as the "healthy diet" came in 1977 when Senator George McGovern and his nutrition committee were trying to address the rise in heart disease in the U.S. Their conclusions were publicized as the Dietary Goals for the United States and would become the Dietary Guidelines for Americans a few years later. Dietary fat and cholesterol were falsely but officially labeled as the cause of heart disease by acommittee of politicians. Opposing views arguing that excess sugar and starch were the real cause of obesity and heart disease were heard but ignored. Since people have to get their energy from somewhere, the shift away from dietary fat led to an increase in the consumption of carbohydrates, especially sugar. Obesity rates have risen ever since, followed by rising rates in Type 2 Diabetes starting 10 years later.

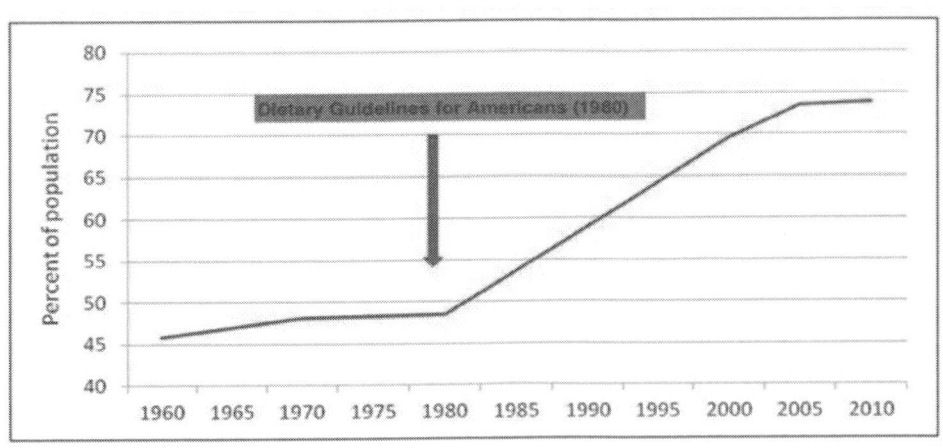

Source: CDC data

Since then, more studies and more careful analysis of previous studies have shown that there is no increased risk associated with total fat, saturated fat or dietary cholesterol intake. A follow up analysis of 21 studies covering over 347,000 patients published in the American Journal of Clinical Nutrition[2] showed that "intake of saturated fat was not associated with an increased risk of CHD, stroke or CVD." The Swedish Malmo Diet and Cancer Study[3] also found that after accounting forthe negative effect of trans fats, neither total dietary fat nor saturated intake showed an increase risk of mortality and the "current dietary guidelines regarding fat intake" were "not supported". One of my personal favorites from Nutrients[4] on dietary cholesterol intake, specifically from eggs found "recent intervention studies with eggs demonstrate that the additional dietary cholesterol does not negatively affect serum lipids, and in some cases, appears to improve lipoprotein particle profiles and HDL functionality." Translation: not only is dietary cholesterol not bad for us but the cholesterol from eggs actually improves our blood cholesterol profile. I find this somewhat validating because I have been eating 3-5 whole eggs a day for over 15 years. No study has ever linked dietary fat with obesity. It was blamed because fat is higher in calories than the other macronutrients but without proof.

In 2016, the Dietary Guidelines for Americans finally backed off of the recommendations to avoid dietary fat and cholesterol but this news didn't receive the same level of attention or marketing that the message to avoid dietary fat and those ever so deadly egg yolks (add sarcastic tone) did for the previous 39 years.

From the Food Comes First 30 Day Weight Loss Facebook Group:

Over the past six years my husband Chris and I have attempted many Diets...low calorie, cutting out carbs, portion control, exercising religiously. Nothing had worked and instead we were both about 50 lbs. overweight. I'm one of those people that if I don't see results right away I loose motivation. When we started the Food Comes First Group we were so ready for a lifestyle change. We had so many epiphanies and breakthrough moments in the 30 days. For me realizing that what food I put in to my body really does matter. In the 30 days I lost 11 lbs. and 2 inches around the belly, and Chris lost 15 lbs., and the best thing is that we don't want to stop! We have a 6 month old baby girl and she is our motivation for a healthy lifestyle. We have so much more energy and for me, not having to wear my maternity clothes anymore is a huge bonus. We love our new healthy lifestyle and couldn't be happier with the changes we have made. Thanks so much Zane!

-Bonnie L., Mesa, AR

CHAPTER 2

LOW CALORIE: HOW LOW CAN YOU GO?

In essence, if we want to direct our lives, we must take control of our consistent actions. It's not what we do once in a while that shapes our lives, but what we do consistently.

-Tony Robbins

The *calorie is a calorie* concept also gave rise to low calorie diets. Essentially, a person's basal or resting metabolic rate (BMR or RMR) is calculated using a formula including their height, weight, age and sex. This is an approximation of the amount of calories the person's body burns in a day at rest. More calories may be added based on their activity level. Then a certain percentage of calories is deducted from that amount as a daily caloric goal for their diet with the idea that the calorie deficit will cause a release of fat for energy from the fat stores, leading to weight loss. For example, let's assume a person's BMR is 2000 cal/day. If you were to reduce caloric intake to 75% of the total BMR which is 1500 cal/day, the expected result would be to burn off 500 cal/day from fat stores.

That is the "scientific" approach you might get from a nutritionist. Many people wanting to lose weight just shootfrom the hip and under eat without the fancy calculations or a "nutritious" reduced calorie diet plan based on the food pyramid shown in chapter 10 recommending 6-11 servings of starches like bread, pasta and cereal *and* 2-4 servings of fruit. They just cut their calories and buy "low calorie" or "fat free" labeled food to get quick results.

As I get older and maybe a little bit wiser, you realize how much stuff affects your body and what it can do. Cutting out carbs and sweets and trying to eat just proteins and fruits and stuff like that, more natural stuff, is what I have found has had the biggest impact on me.

-Jay Cutler, NFL Quarterback

Makes sense doesn't it? Except that our bodies don't act like a linear 6th grade math problem. You will hear proponents of low calorie diets quote the law of thermodynamics saying that the energy we burn off has to come from somewhere. This assertion is based on the assumption that our basal metabolic rate and other uses of energy don't change or adjust to accommodate the amount of food we eat.

Exercise only accounts for about 5-10% of our total energy burned. Maintaining normal body functions takes up the majority of our energy needs with the greatest amount of energy used coming from our brain, heart, liver and kidneys, all of which is out of our conscious control. The energy needs of these organs can vary depending on whether we're asleep, we've just eaten or we're under some kind of stress.

What would happen if the body continued to expend 3000 calories daily while taking in only 1500? Soon fat stores would be burned, then protein stores would be burned, and then you would die. Nice. The smart course of action for the body is to immediately reduce caloric expenditure to 1500 calories per day to restore balance.

-Jason Fung, M.D., Author

For example, our body temperature can fluctuate for several reasons but it is controlled by hormones, just like our metabolism, heart rate, energy levels, and many other bodily functions. Of the six people in our family, three are female. My wife, who is my age, and our two daughters who are in their late teens and early twenties. Despite the fact that the room temperature hasn't budged from 69 degrees, body temperatures in our household can vary greatly and hour to hour. You would think we were subject to arctic blasts and desert winds regardless of the season.

Of course this couldn't possibly be the result of recent changes in caloric intake, activity level or "other" hormonal fluctuations which can affect the generation of body heat. It *must* be a problem with the thermostat which requires an immediate and dramatic adjustment to the temperature setting.

Since we have a two story house with separate thermostats for each floor there have been times when a thermodynamic battle has ensued between the warm air from the heat that is on downstairs which rises to turn on the cool air from the A/C upstairs and vice versa.

The upstairs thermostat set to cool will have to come on more often to counter the effect of the warm air rising from downstairs in order to maintain the temperature it is set to. Clearly, it wouldn't have to come on as often to maintain its temperature setting if the heater wasn't on downstairs. It seems obvious, right? You can't have a source of warm air and a source of cool air operating in the same house without them having some effect on each other, essentially one being signaled to cancel out the effect of the other.

Our bodies have a very similar relationship with the amount of energy we eat, the amount that we burn and the body weight set point it is trying to maintain. When there is a consistent reduction of available energy (food) over an extended period of time, our brain realizes that this can't continue if it is going to maintain the body weight set point. This is part of the process of maintaining homeostasis.

The low calorie diet can cause a short term drop in weight but eventually the body won't be able to keep up with this energy shortage at the current level of basal metabolism, activity level and body heat, so it adapts. Using hormones, the hypothalamus signals the body to reduce the basal metabolic rate so you don't starve to death. It is fighting against the effects of the low fat, low calorie diet to maintain the set point. In addition to reducing the energy used to keep our organs working, maintain our activity levels and reduce heat production it also signals the release of more hunger producing hormones like ghrelin. The result is lower energy, decreased body temperature so we may feel cold, increased hunger, slowed weight loss and we probably aren't much fun to be around.

This also leads to what is called "yo-yo dieting". Eventually we get tired of being hungry and lethargic and return to our previous level of eating but our metabolic rate has slowed so we put the weight right back on, and sometimes a bit more.

From the Food Comes First 30 Day Weight Loss Facebook Group:

I just completed Zane's 30 day weight loss group. I lost 11 lbs., and over 5" combined from my waist, hips, and chest. And, that's not even the good news! You know how you count down the days 'til a "30 day diet" is over? Day 31 came and went and I honestly forgot it was over. I WANTED to keep going. This is hands-down the easiest weight I've ever lost. I enjoyed every single meal, and I gained so much knowledge of what to eat.

-Jen S., Franklin, TN

CHAPTER 3

WE ARE NOT ALONE...

When something is important enough, you do it even if the odds are not in your favor.

-Elon Musk

An incredibly overlooked component of weight control and our overall health is our microbiome. The recently revised number of bacteria in our microbiome is approximately 30-50 trillion. Our biome also includes trillions of viruses, fungi and other microbes in addition to the bacteria living in and on our bodies. There are approximately 30 trillion cells in the human body, so in a sense, we are outnumbered. These organisms are in constant communication with our cells and actually make up the bulk of our immune system, as well as control many other functions in our bodies. We couldn't live without them.

Have you ever heard of a poop transplant? Yes, I said poop. They take the poop from a person with a very healthy biome and transplant it into the bowel of a person who needs to improve their biome, usually struggling to lose weight. Yes, it works. Clinics in Europe have been performing the procedure for decades. There is actually a clinician in the United States who is making capsules containing freeze dried poop from a carefully selected group of donors with impeccable diets and using them as supplements to treat patients.

Generally, in the U.S. the procedure is used to treat a bacterial infection that causes diarrhea and can be fatal but the procedure can also be used to reverse obesity and improve insulin sensitivity.

The type of bacteria we have living in our biome determines which diseases we get, our mental state and, more to the point, our weight. More than 90% of the bacteria in the gut is made up of two different groups: **Firmicutes** and **Bacteroidetes**.

Firmicutes are very efficient at extracting energy from food. In other words, if you have a high population of Firmicutes, you would absorb more calories from the food you eat than someone with a smaller population of those bacteria. According to research, obese people tend to have more Firmicutes than Bacteroidetes, whereas lean people have a larger population of Bacteroidetes than Firmicutes. The ratio of these two types of bacteria is called the **F/B ratio**. Higher levels of Firmicutes can actually cause a greater expression of the genes that increase the risk of obesity, cardiovascular disease and diabetes.

How do I change my F/B ratio?

You're probably asking HOW you can change your F/B ratio and make sure you have the right balance of bacteria in your body to control your weight and avoid disease. It turns out that we can greatly affect the population of our biomes with how we eat.

In 2010, a Harvard study[5] compared the stool samples of children from two different populations of people and found that people living in rural Africa who eat a lot of vegetable fiber have higher amounts of Bacteroidetes than people living in Europe with greater access to processed, starchy and sugary food, who have a higher population of Firmicutes (a higher F/B ratio). In both cases, the dominant bacteria outnumbered the other by 2 to 1. The F/B ratio is actually being considered an obesity biomarker.

It appears that Bacteroidetes grow when the diet is made up of non-starchy vegetables like asparagus, Brussels sprouts, broccoli, greens, cabbage, green beans, onions, garlic, artichokes, sprouts and other bulky plant fiber.

Firmicuties, which are dominant in overweight people, flourish when the diet contains starchy and sugary food. These are foods that are more easily digested and turned into energy. These bacteria also impact genes that affect metabolism and make the body think it needs to hold on to calories. Yikes! They affect insulin sensitivity and inflammation, symptoms we try to control with medicines but often without addressing our diet.

Fortunately, most people can change their F/B ratio without requiring a poop transplant. We just have to feed the type of bacteria we want with the foods they like to eat and that provide a healthy environment for them to grow. as well as avoid the foods that inflame their environment and feed the bacteria we do not want to grow.

If you have seen any of my videos on Facebook or YouTube then you know what I am about to say. We need to follow a low carb, high fat diet that is full of non-starchy vegetables, which cause the Bacteroidetes to flourish.

Just to clarify, I am not talking about the typical low carb, high fat diet that includes large amounts of processed protein and fat with little focus on vegetables and fruit. Obviously we need lots of vegetable fiber to feed a healthy biome. Processed foods, including processed protein and fat as well as carbs, cause inflammation in our bodies and in particular, our gut.

The purpose of this diet is to reverse the cycle of insulin resistance and fat storage and create an environment for improved insulin sensitivity, fat release and fat burning metabolism. To do this, we have to look beyond calories and even macronutrients (fat, protein, carbs) and eat a diet that creates a healthy biome because of its influence over our metabolism. If our F/B ratio affects how much energy we absorb from the food we eat and how much we release to be burned for fuel then doesn't it make sense to make improving it a focus of the way we eat?

I'm trying to do the paleo diet. No carbs.
-Robin Wright, Actress

Why don't we hear more about our biome in the health and fitness media?

The effect and importance of our biome is an extremely progressive study and most of the mainstream health and medical community don't know much about it. If you are interested in learning more about the biome, I highly recommend two books by Dr. David Perlmutter: "Grain Brain" and "Brain Maker". Dr. Perlmutter, a neurologist motivated to prevent diseases of the brain, looked to nutrition for answers and found that what is good for the brain is good for the whole body as well.

From the Food Comes First 30 Day Weight Loss Facebook Group:

Thanks for this, Zane. Thanks for the support of the group. I learned a lot about this weight loss process through FCF. I've gone from almost clueless to clumsily capable. I would put my weight loss at about 10 pounds. (I had to buy a new scale during week 1) I believe that I've lost a pant size. I guess what I'm happiest aboutis the feeling of having some control over my diet. It's more about vigilance than deprivation. That makes this seem like a long term plan. I'll probably drop in on a group a few months later for a refresher...

-Danny Wilburn, Gadsden, AL

CHAPTER 4

HIGH FAT, LOW CARB

You are a clay sculpture, a work of art, being formed by the trials of each day…and God isn't finished with you yet.
                                                                -Anonymous

Most people are familiar with the idea of a low carb diet. It's when I say "high fat" that I get the question marks. We have been conditioned through over 40 years of incorrect dietary guidelines to be afraid of dietary fat.

There are some fats that we should avoid and I will talk about those but naturally occurring fats like those in meat, eggs, poultry, nuts, seeds, avocados, coconut oil, butter or any other dairy and olive oil are not to be feared. In fact, the fat from these sources should make up the majority of the energy we eat. You'll notice that list is a mix of saturated, polyunsaturated and monounsaturated fats.

Fat provides twice as much energy, or calories, per gram as carbohydrates AND has little to no effect on the release of insulin. This makes it a great replacement for starchy and sugary carbs because it will stay in our system longer, giving us satiety and a consistent supply of energy, and it won't inhibit the release of fat from our fat stores.

The idea that saturated fat was bad for us destroyed our relationship with food.
    –Dr. Cate Shanahan, M.D., Nutrition Advisor for the L.A. Lakers, Author

Those are also the reasons we don't have to be on a low calorie diet to lose weight BUT may end up eating less naturally, without hunger and without signaling to reduce our metabolic rate. The ups and downs of insulin and other hormones that come with eating starch and sugars stimulate hunger and can lead to cravings and excessive snacking, usually on more carbs. The low carb diet described in this book allows for more of our stored fat to be burned, therefore we can supplement more of our energy needs from our fat stores and the hypothalamus does not get the signal that we're starving so our metabolic rate stays up.

If you're looking for some mainstream medical affirmation about the benefits of a low carb, high fat diet, you can check out a Harvard study published in the Journal of the American Medical Association (JAMA) in June, 2012 titled, "Effects of Dietary Composition on Energy Expenditure during Weight-Loss Maintenance".[6] The study put overweight or obese young adults on three different diets for a month: a low fat diet consisting of 60% carb, 20% fat and 20% protein; a low glycemic diet consisting of 40% carbs, 40% fat and 20% protein; and a low carb diet consisting of 10% carb, 60% fat and 30% protein. All of the diets contained the same number of calories. The people on the low carb diet burned the most calories and had the most improvement in insulin sensitivity, almost twice as much improvement of insulin sensitivity as the people on the low fat diet. Those on the low fat diet also showed changes in blood chemistry that would make them more likely to have weight gain. The conclusion was that the low carb, high fat diet was the best one for maintaining weight loss. So much for "a calorie is a calorie".

From my Facebook fitness page: facebook.com/zanesblog

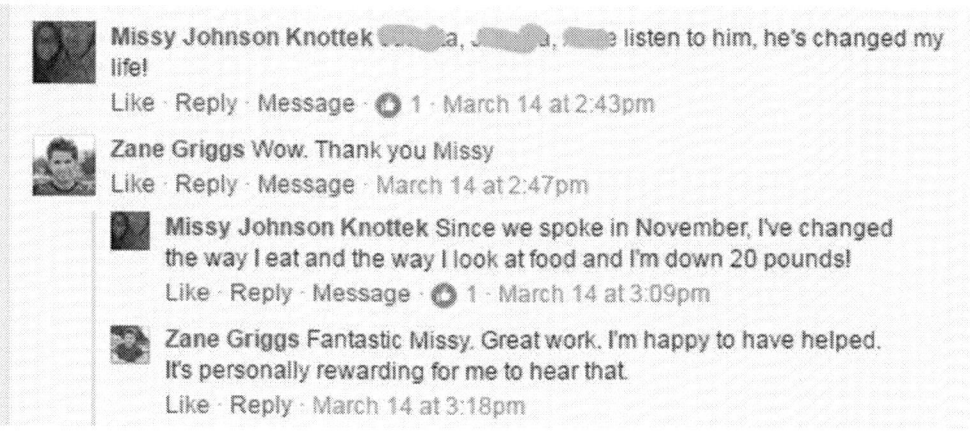

Making the switch to fat

Making the switch to fat as your primary energy source when you have been used to a high carb diet requires an adaptation in your body's metabolism. Many people experience a 2-3 week adjustment period while their fat burning metabolism becomes more efficient at producing energy. This adjustment period has been called the "carb flu" because some people will experience energy swings and even headaches as their body makes this shift, in many cases breaking an addiction to sugar and instigating some cleansing to take place.

If you experience some of these symptoms, DO NOT QUIT! It is not a "sign" that this isn't the plan for you. It's more likely a sign that you are too dependent on carbohydrates for your daily energy. As mentioned before, talk to your healthcare provider and keep them in the loop, especially if you have medical concerns or have been treated regarding your blood sugar regulation.

The idea of it is you train your body to burn healthy fats and so I eat healthy fats all day long.

-Halle Berry, Actress

Fats to avoid...

There are some fats we want to avoid because they cause inflammation in our bodies. Inflammation causes cell damage, which is the beginning stages of disease and aging. Everyone, including the government health authorities, agrees that trans fats should be avoided. These are the hydrogenated or partially hydrogenated oils we see as ingredients in many packaged foods. This is a man-made process used to make the unsaturated fats added to the food last longer on the shelf. You'll see oils like hydrogenated cottonseed oil or soybean oil listed in so many foods like non-dairy creamers, cereals, breads, margarine, snack foods and desserts.

These trans fats which were at one time called the healthy alternative to naturally occurring saturated fat have since been shown to increase the risk of heart disease and stroke. as well as raise LDL cholesterol and lower HDL cholesterol. Many of the studies, like the Framingham study[7], that had pointed to saturated fat as the cause for heart disease, after closer scrutiny, showed that it was the trans fats, which are artificial saturated fats, like margarine that had increased the risk of heart disease and raised LDL cholesterol. Additionally, the naturally occurring saturated fats like butter or other animal fats, had no relation to heart disease.

Vegetable oils are toxic and compose anywhere from 30%-60% of the calories in the standard American diet.
  –Dr. Cate Shanahan, M.D., Nutrition Advisor for the L.A. Lakers, Author

The other fats to avoid are cooking oils like canola oil, corn oil and safflower oil which are liquid at room temperature. These are polyunsaturated fats, which we have been told to use for cooking for decades now. The problem with cooking with these oils is that unsaturated fats have a low smoke point, which means they oxidize at high heat. Oxidation is like rust and it causes cell damage and inflammation in our bodies. Polyunsaturated fats are good to eat when in a whole food like nuts and fish but not after they've been extracted and processed as a cooking oil. Unlike extra virgin olive oil which is extracted by crushing the olives, these oils are extracted using heat and chemicals which damages the oils causing oxidation to begin immediately after extraction.

When eating at restaurants, avoid eating foods that have been cooked in a fryer. They are generally using these same polyunsaturated vegetable oils at high heat and many times the oil is only changed once a week or even two weeks. The longer the oil is used the more oxidized it becomes.

What about olive oil?

Olive oil is a monounsaturated fat like the majority of the fat in avocados. Its smoke point is higher than the other cooking oils but because its unsaturated (liquid at room temperature) it is not as stable as a saturated fat so it will oxidize when used for cooking. As mentioned before, look for extra virgin olive oil which is extracted through the physical crushing of the olive rather than the use of heat or chemicals. If you really must use it for cooking occasionally, keep the temperature very low. The best use for olive oil is as a dressing on salads. It is a very healthy fat to consume as long as it has not been oxidized.

Stable fats for cooking are natural saturated fats like coconut oil, butter, duck fat, beef tallow and ghee. If you are still concerned about saturated fats causing an increased risk of heart disease, I suggest two books written by cardiologists that helped me have a better understanding of what really causes cardiovascular disease...and what doesn't.

1. **The Cure for Heart Disease** by Dwight Lundell and Todd R. Nordstrom
2. **The Great Cholesterol Myth** by Jonny Bowden and Stephen Sinatra

From week 3 of the Food Comes First 30 Day Weight Loss Facebook Group:

I first connected with Zane in November of 2016. I learned so much from him, changed so many of my habits and lost 25 pounds! But, I let 'life' get the best of me and slipped into some old eating habits. Fast forward to April 2018, unhealthy and tipped the scales at 223 lbs. I saw a picture of myself and said "I'm done". It was so easy to pick back up what Zane taught me. From May to December, I was down 35 pounds! Since the planner, this group support and cutting the carbs and sugars, I'm down another 8 pounds! Everything I've learned has gotten me to where I am and I couldn't be more grateful. The struggles, the healthy choices vs. the unhealthy are working (though some days it's not easy!)

-Missy Knottek, Ottawa, Illinois

CHAPTER 5

OBESITY IS A FORM OF INTERNAL STARVATION

And you ask 'What if I fall?' Oh but my darling, what if you fly?
—Erin Hanson

Isn't that a head scratcher? The fear of dietary fat led to the rise of low fat and low calorie diets. Both of these diets would be considered high carb diets because at least 50% of the calories come from carbohydrates. The problem is that a high carb diet can lead to insulin resistance in which calories are quickly swept out of the bloodstream, passed the resistant muscle cells and into the fat cells. The presence of insulin, especially the elevated insulin levels resulting from insulin resistance, keeps excess fat locked up in the fat cells. This gives the fat cells priority over the muscles, brain and other organs in the body. That's right! Insulin pushes the energy into the fat cells before the other tissues are properly fed.

As a result, the brain triggers a starvation response because it doesn't see all of the calories locked up in the fat cells. It just knows that calories are being used up too quickly so it sends signals to **lower the metabolic rate AND increase the appetite**. The result is that we create less energy, we're lethargic and, if that wasn't bad enough, we're HUNGRY! Can you see how the internal starvation cycle could make someone obese? It's not about the *amount* of calories being eaten that begins the process. It's the *type* of calories.

In addition to this, other stress hormones are elevated like cortisol and epinephrine which creates inflammation, causes harmful effects on our heart and arteries, and causes us to break down muscle in a fight or flight state.

Now, we see ourselves gaining weight on this low fat, high carb diet and what is our typical response? We cut calories. Without changing the type of calories we're eating, we just reduce the number and increase the starvation response even more. We have more hunger and an even lower metabolic rate while the calories continue to be shuttled to the fat cells because of insulin resistance.

OBESITY IS NOT caused by an excess of calories, but instead by a body set weight that is too high because of a hormonal imbalance in the body.
-Jason Fung, M.D., Author

The hypothalamus has a weight "set point" as mentioned earlier which it recognizes as the weight your body is supposed to be. You may not agree with that set point but the survival response in your brain will do whatever it takes to maintain that set point. The set point weight can change over time but you can see how it is not going to work out too well with a low fat, low calorie diet.

This is a great example of how our weight and body fat are regulated by hormones, not calories. The set point is can be very much affected by insulin resistance when present. The hypothalamus can reduce the metabolic rate, reduce body heat production and release hunger producing hormones in an effort to maintain the body weight set point to counter any reduction of calories. In my opinion, reducing insulin resistance and therefore the amount of insulin in the bloodstream is the best way change the set point and release more body fat for energy.

You may have seen the news story about the former *The Biggest Loser* participants who have gained much or all of their previous weight back.[8] There was an observational study which kept track of several of them to see how they did after the show. The big news from the study was that many of them had a metabolic rate that was 300-400 calories a day lower than a person of similar height, age, weight and the same sex would have. This shocked and discouraged a lot of people. The study really didn't provide a good explanation for it either.

Basically, their bodies were trying to gain the weight back and return to a particular set point. Why? If we consider the previously mentioned issues with low fat, high carb diets and low calorie diets we might assume that the stress of 6- 8 hours of exercise a day, being underfed for their size and activity level and that what they did eat was based on a typical low fat diet, this plan did not allow for their set point to decrease with their rapid loss of bodyweight. The protection against starvation was still in place.

Add the 300-400 cal/day lower metabolism to a return to a normal life with all of its responsibilities, a moderate activity level, a much less strict diet, and *without* the dramatics of a celebrity trainer shouting in their face and you have the formula for weight gain.

From the Food Comes First Weight Loss Group:

I'm so happy I decided to join your Food Comes First weight loss group. It was so worth it. You make sense about what to eat and when. I know now when my body is fat adapted and when I follow your plan, the pounds come off. Plus, I have more energy and sleep better at night. I now have fewer "eaters remorse" meals. While in your group I lost 15 lbs. in 6 weeks and I'm keeping it off. I'm planning on losing another 20 lbs. I encourage anyone to join your next challenge group. Blessings to you for continuing helping people in their weight loss goals.

-Amy Hickok, Bakersfield, CA

CHAPTER 6

INTERMITTENT FASTING

Worry does not empty tomorrow of its sorrow, it empties today of its strength.

-Corrie Boom

Please don't let that "F" word scare you. Fasting has had a bad reputation in the fitness industry but it is actually a great technique to increase and improve fat burning. I'm including this section about intermittent fasting (IF) as an *option* because it is so effective but it is not mandatory. Intermittent fasting, or time restricted eating as it is also called, simply adds more hours during which your body has to rely on burning stored fat for fuel.

The basics of good nutrition can be summarized in these simple rules. Eat whole, unprocessed foods. Avoid sugar. Avoid refined grains. Eat a diet high in natural fats. Balance feeding with fasting.

-Jason Fung, M.D., Author

There are several ways to practice IF. I will cover two of the more popular methods here. The first is to do 24-36 hour fasts each week. Some people may do this once or twice a week and others may fast every other day while eating sufficient calories on the non-fasting days which helps keep the basal metabolic rate from dropping. The second method is to restrict eating each day to an eight hour window, allowing 16 hours for fasting, only drinking water, black coffee or plain tea during the fasting period. No cream or sweeteners, including artificial sweeteners which still elevate insulin despite containing no calories.

The second method using the eight hour eating window is not meant to be a low calorie diet. You can still eat a sufficient amount of calories in the eight hour window. As an example, you might eat your first meal at 12:00 pm, a second around 3:00 or 4:00 pm and dinner at 7:00 but stop eating at 8:00 pm until the next day at 12:00 pm.

The body enters a fasted state about 12 hours after eating the last meal so this plan puts the body in a fasted state for four hours each day. This not only increases the amount of fat burning but also trains the body to burn fat more efficiently and improves insulin sensitivity.

I like to gently introduce this method to the Food Comes First 30 Day Weight Loss Group on an optional basis. For those who are open, we compress the eating time to eight hours, every other day, for a week making four intermittent fasting days with their usual schedule staggered between them.

Facebook post from the Food Comes First 30 Day Weight Loss Group:

> **Rose Marie Smith** 'Win.. focused while on vacation'...
> I've been on vacation for 8 days in non-the-less than Las Vegas and California... The smells of any kind of food everywhere! I have been able to stick to my daily intermittent fasting.. I haven't had access to a scale this whole time, but I made great choices the whole time.. and lots of walking! So we shall see if there has been changes tonight when I get back to TN.

> **Rose Marie Smith** Update...
> I lost 2 lbs while on vacation!!.. What? That never happens to me... Thank you Zane Griggs your tools are easy to keep in my head and follow...

The first two weeks of intermittent fasting will require some discipline as your body adjusts to relying more on fat stores for fuel. Feeling hungry is nothing to be afraid of. That growling in your stomach is actually a hormonal response to a lower blood sugar level but it won't hurt you. Just ignore it, or drink some water, and it will likely stop in 10 or 15 minutes. Many people find that once their bodies adjust to the new schedule, their energy levels are more consistent and they are quite happy to start their day with some black coffee or tea and without the trouble of preparing and eating breakfast.

There are other health benefits to fasting besides weight loss and improved insulin sensitivity like the recycling of damaged cells, called autophagy, and improved brain health. Medically supervised fasting is being used to treat and reverse many diseases like Type 2 Diabetes, auto-immune diseases and even cancer in integrative medicine treatments and in therapeutic fasting centers like TrueNorth in California and Buchinger-Wilhelmi in Europe. If you would like more information on these benefits I highly recommend checking out the research of Dr. Mark Mattson at the National Institute on Aging and the Johns Hopkins University School of Medicine.

If your goal is to increase fat burning, whether to just lean out a bit or to lose a significant amount of weight, the combination of a low carb diet with either approach to intermittent fasting is a powerful technique for getting the body to use stored fat without starving it of the calories it needs and causing the metabolic problems that come with low fat, low calorie diets. If you are diabetic or being treated for high blood sugar, high blood pressure or any other medical condition, you will need to consult with your doctor before beginning any fasting regimen to work with you on adjusting medications and monitoring your condition. Please do not ignore this warning. Fasting can be a very effective method for losing weight but if you are being treated for any condition you will need to work with a physician to integrate fasting with your treatment.

From the Food Comes First 30 Day Weight Loss Facebook Group:

So I started the Food Comes First in January 2019. Over the years I had gained a lot of weight, and by the time I was 46 years old I was EXTREMELY overweight. The clothes in my closet didn't fit and I felt dumpy and yuck! I had tried various weight loss plans over the years and had some success, but always gained the weight back, plus more. My sister encouraged me to try this new plan with Zane, she and I would do it together. Although I never thought I would be successful on a low carb plan, I bought the book and jumped on board. The first few days were tough, I really experienced the "Carb Flu", but through Zane's encouragement I battled through. After the first week, my hunger really subsided and my energy was up. I continued to watch the scale move and this was extremely motivating to me! Actual weekly results!

I participated in the intermittent fasting challenge and that really helped the weight loss. The fasting was A LOT easier than I thought it would be. I really thought I would die without eating breakfast! But it really worked for me and became a very easy tool to help with my weight loss.

Over the 4 weeks, I lost a total of 14.5 pounds. The first 30 days all I did was focus on what was going in my mouth. Learning to read labels and make better choices. Learning that a healthy choice doesn't just mean I have to eat salad all the time.

Being overweight most of my adult life, I finally decided this was the year I was going to do something about it. I lost my dad in August 2017 to Lou Gehrig's disease at the age of 70. I slowly watched him lose his ability to walk, speak and care for himself. This made me take a step back and really take a look at my health, to place value on my health. Made me really think about what I was putting in my body and the potential harm I could be doing to my longevity. I plan to continue on with the plan until I achieve my goal. Zane's plan and support has made it plain and simple to understand, which is exactly what I needed. He encourages even when we make the wrong choice. So helpful to have his support and support of the group!

-Kerry Smith, Madera, CA

CHAPTER 7

WHAT ABOUT EXERCISE?

Be miserable. Or motivate yourself. Whatever has to be done, it's always your choice.

-Wayne Dyer

Exercise is certainly an important component to overall health and weight loss. It actually improves your biome as well.

As a trainer and as someone who has been working out regularly since I was 17, I know that exercise is a crucial component of physical and mental health. It is NOT the secret to weight loss. Unless you are training several hours a day like a competitive athlete (or a *The Biggest Loser* participant) your workout will most likely burn an extra 200-300 calories a day- around 10% of your total calories burned for the day. That amount can be easily replaced with what we eat throughout the day, particularly since exercise increases appetite. If you're rewarding yourself after working out with sweetened yogurt, a smoothie full of fruit and whatever so called "healthy" sweetener they use or some other sweet treat, you're probably going in the opposite direction.

As I mentioned earlier, I had the opportunity to work as a trainer with one of the popular weight loss shows called *Extreme Weight Loss* on two seasons, basically putting the participants through workouts five days a week, helping them manage their diet, monitoring weigh ins, and generally staying in touch all the time for support while they were living at home. Even when they were exercising 4-5 hours a day, five days a week, when the diet was off they didn't lose weight, or at least what was expected by a large degree.

Essentially, you cannot out exercise a bad diet which is why I say **food comes first**. I would recommend getting your eating plan in place first and then making adjustments to it as needed to work with your exercise plan.

We've all heard the advertisements for weight loss plans saying you can still "eat the foods you love" as if changing your diet isn't necessary. To me, that's like saying you can graduate from college without studying. Sure there are some gifted individuals who can do it but it is not true for most people. Even if this were the case for someone in their teens or twenties, as we get older we become less sensitive to insulin and exercise alone does not produce the same effect on fat loss.

This pyramid shows the priority I recommend for success with weight loss starting with diet at the base and the first in importance, followed by sleep which I will cover in the next chapter and then three types of exercise which I will go over in this chapter. Since both fat storage and fat release are regulated primarily by hormones, rather than pure caloric expenditure, these are in order of influence on the hormones that effect fat storage.

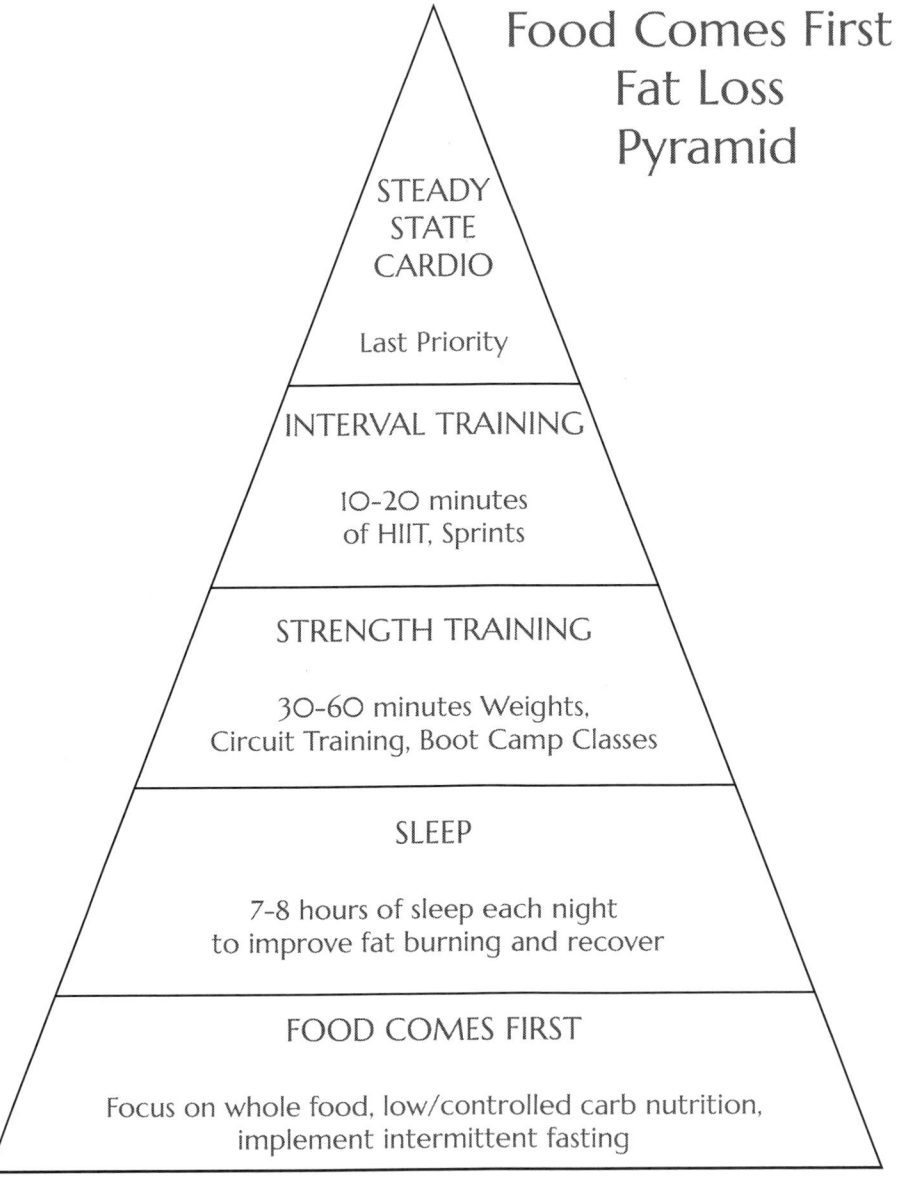

Resistance Training

Strength training is effective for improving insulin sensitivity and increasing fat loss. Resistance training reduces the amount of glycogen, or energy, stored in the muscle, which signals the body to replace this energy from food recently eaten and/or from fat and liver stores. As I mentioned before, insulin resistance is when muscle cells are no longer sensitive to insulin and don't allow more fuel to be stored in them, causing insulin to store the fuel in the fat cells instead. Insulin sensitivity is improved when the stored glycogen is used and the body is signaled to store more fuel in the muscles.

The exercise sets should be intense enough to cause the muscle to fatigue or hit failure in less than 2 minutes, which is usually between 5 and 20 repetitions. Burning off stored glycogen is also specific to the muscles being trained so resistance training for the legs will not affect the muscles in the upper body. A 20 minute steady state cardio session will not be as effective at improving insulin sensitivity as a fast paced, 20 minute, full body resistance training session.

Note: when I refer to "post workout carbs" in the plan, the type of workout I am referring to is some kind of resistance training like lifting weights, a boot camp style class or bodyweight based movements rather than a cardio workout.

I know that many people trying to lose weight, especially women, are concerned that weight training will cause them to gain weight. Generally speaking, most women do not have enough testosterone to unintentionally put on a lot of muscle weight. In fact, most men over 30 struggle to put on muscle even when they are trying to. Bodybuilding requires a person to perform very intense and frequent workouts focusing on specific muscle groups at each session. In contrast, circuit training two or three days a week is not an effective routine for building muscle mass. Over feeding, or eating more calories than burned, is usually necessary for significant muscle growth and the diet is generally a high carb diet.

Weight loss statistics show that an average of 25% of weight loss is muscle weight. This is not ideal. We want to lose fat, not muscle. Resistance training can help the body retain muscle weight during weight loss by signaling the body to store more glycogen in the muscle. Essentially, use it or lose it.

Is it possible that you *may* gain a few pounds of muscle from resistance training over time? Yes, but think of it this way. The fuel you store in your muscles has to go somewhere. Would you rather that it is stored as muscle or as fat? Keep in mind that 2 to 3 pounds of muscle is A LOT smaller than 2 to 3 pounds of fat and burns twice as much energy at rest.

If your goal is weight loss and you are consistently losing weight, it is very difficult to gain any muscle and you are likely to lose some muscle rather than gain it, even if you are resistance training.

I have found that circuit training is a great way to get a full workout done in a shorter period of time. By circuit training, I mean moving through a series of exercises working different muscles so that while you are working one group, the others are resting. For example, you could do a set of an upper body exercise, then a lower body exercise, followed by a core exercise with little to no rest between sets for two to four rounds and then move on to a new circuit.

An example of this kind of circuit would be 3 sets of each of the following:
Circuit 1: Squat, Chest Press, Leg Lift
Circuit 2: Lunge, Row, Plank
Circuit 3: Hip Bridges, Overhead Press, Reverse Crunch

Doing all three circuits three times each would be a total of 27 sets. Keeping a consistent pace, you could get a full body workout completed in 20 to 40 minutes. This could be performed 2 or 3 times a week, essentially every other day, allowing at least one day off from resistance training between workouts since it is a full body workout. It could be followed by your cardio workout or your cardio could be done later that day or on the alternate days between the resistance workouts depending on your schedule.

If you need to do your resistance training on consecutive days, splitting your muscle groups into two different workouts is a good idea. For example you could work your upper body on Monday and your lower body and core on Tuesday. I would still allow a day off from resistance training after those two consecutive workout days. In this example, you could skip resistance training on Wednesday to rest or just do some cardio, and do the same type of workout split on Thursday and Friday. You could alternately do a full body circuit on Thursday and a non-resistance training workout on Friday like cardio or yoga. There are many ways to make it work with your schedule, mix it up and get it done.

Cardiovascular Training

In my opinion, cardiovascular exercise has been over used and abused, often as a way to work off a bad dietary decision. Am I saying that cardiovascular exercise isn't helpful? No, I'm not saying that at all. In my experience and from what I have studied, cardio training is most effective for weight loss when used at certain times in combination with a low carb diet and resistance training as a way to train the fat burning metabolic system to work more efficiently, rather than as a way to just burn off extra calories.

Training the fat burning system to work more efficiently will help you to burn fat more efficiently throughout your day even when you are not exercising and to be less reliant on carbs for energy, especially when combined with a low carb diet. Your energy levels will be steadier and you will have fewer cravings for carbs.

Fat burning metabolism, the release and burning of stored fat, uses a different system than glycogen burning metabolism, glycogen being the predominant fuel stored in muscles. Using glycogen is a much faster supply of energy and is what our bodies use first for more intense activity. We want our bodies to be efficient at burning both types of fuel in appropriate ratios. This is called metabolic flexibility. For instance, you would not want your body to be primarily burning glycogen while sitting on the couch or driving your car. Ideally we want our bodies to be primarily burning stored fat during low intensity activities.

One of the more effective times to do cardio for weight loss is right after a resistance training session when glycogen stores in the muscles are low.

Another very effective time for a cardio workout to train the fat burning metabolism is when you are in a fasted state. By fasted state, I mean before you have eaten any calories that day, whether that's first thing in the morning or at noon. Drinking water, black coffee or tea (no cream or sugar) is fine and even recommended, but consume no food or liquid that would add calories for fuel to be burned during the workout. This will cause the body to rely more on your fat burning metabolism. If you need to perform your cardio later in the day after you have already begun eating, try to allow at least two hours after your last meal before beginning the cardio session to make the most of lower blood sugar levels.

The energy supply from fat burning is slower. Because of this you may not be able to work out as fast or for as long as you would if you had eaten before the workout. The point is to train the fat burning metabolic system to work more efficiently rather than to just burn off calories or have a stronger workout. A 20 to 40 minute cardio session is enough to be effective for training the system but not overdo it.

My recommended meal after a cardio workout would be 20-40 grams of protein, fat and perhaps some non-starchy vegetables but would not include starchy carbohydrates. Since the primary purpose of this workout is to improve your fat burning metabolism, allow your body to replace energy with body fat or dietary fat rather than refueling with carbs.

Doing too much cardio can cause an increase in appetite and even cravings for quick energy supplying carbs. Be careful not to increase it to the point that you are sabotaging your eating plan. Training for a half marathon or other long distance event would not be my recommendation *if your reason for doing so is to lose weight.* You might find that when you're doing an hour or more of cardio at a time that you will start craving more carbs than you had been eating previously. It can also increase inflammation in muscles, joints, etc. which may cause a craving for comfort foods. This is counterproductive *if weight loss is your goal.*

When I'm training for 'True Blood,' I don't eat any sugar except for some fruit here and there. So it's no sugar, no bread, no real carbs all day

-Joe Manganiello, Actor

Steady State vs. High Intensity Interval Training

The most common form of cardio is steady state cardio in which you move at a pace during which the energy needed can be maintained primarily by aerobic energy production. Generally speaking if you can maintain the pace for five minutes or more, it is primarily aerobic.

High intensity interval training (HIIT) involves alternating intervals of the movement at a faster pace for 30 seconds to 2 minutes with a slower recovery pace of about the same duration. The higher intensity interval is at a faster pace than aerobic energy alone can maintain and causes lactic acid to build up in the muscle. This type of cardio challenges the upper limits of the cardiovascular system, as well as the fat burning metabolic system and burns off more stored glycogen in the muscle than steady state cardio.

Both types of cardio training can be used effectively and I personally use both in my routine. You and your healthcare provider can decide which is best for you.

When fat burning is the goal, I do not recommend eating right before resistance or cardio training. A pre-workout meal will improve performance during the workout but it is likely to inhibit fat burning.

From the Food Comes First 30 Day Weight Loss Facebook Group:

I have lost 9.8 lbs. in total during the 30 days of your program... I'm still working it, however I do miss the daily coaching...this has all the elements of so many things I have read through the years, but you have simplified it so that I think this can definitely be a way of life.

-Rose Smith, Fairview, TN

CHAPTER 8

WHEN IS THE BEST TIME TO EAT CARBS?

Never lower your target; increase your actions.
                                               -Grant Cardone

This approach may also be the opposite of what you have been told before. On this plan, starchy carbs are eaten at the end of the day with or after dinner. This is because of hormones that are released in our bodies at different times of the day.

Our bodies work on a cycle with our sympathetic and para-sympathetic nervous systems, collectively known as the autonomic nervous system[9]. In the morning and throughout our day, the sympathetic nervous system releases hormones like adrenaline and epinephrine to wake us up and give us energy to be active. These hormones are also conducive to releasing fat if insulin is not elevated. In the evening, our para-sympathetic nervous system begins to take over releasing hormones like serotonin and melatonin to help us relax and prepare for sleep and recovery.

We have all experienced that drop in energy a couple of hours after eating a large serving of starch or sugar. We generally feel a bit tired because insulin has swept away the fuel from our bloodstream to store it in muscle or fat cells. Not only does this cause energy swings during what should be our most productive hours but it also inhibits fat burning when we are the most primed for it.

Increase your consumption of healthful fats like extra virgin olive oil, avocado, grass-fed beef, wild fish, coconut oil, nuts and seeds. At the same time, keep in mind that modified fats like hydrogenated or trans fats are the worst choices for brain health.
-David Perlmutter, M.D., Neurologist, Author

We can take advantage of the adrenaline boosted, active part of our day to burn body fat by keeping insulin levels low and eating non-starchy veggies, protein and fat. Starchy carbs are great for refueling and recovery so by eating them in the evening we are working with the hormones that help us recover from our day and get into a deeper sleep.

As I mentioned before, the exception to this would be after an intense workout that empties the glycogen stored in our muscles. If you are just doing a moderate cardio workout, you can certainly eat a recovery meal but try not to eat any starchy or sugary carbs to let your fat burning metabolism keep working to help you recover. If you are doing some kind of resistance training, intense boot camp style class or something that had your muscles fatiguing and requiring rest about 30 seconds to 2 minutes into the particular exercise movement or set and you feel like you need a little extra help recovering, you can eat a half of a serving, about 15 grams, of carbs or less. This could be a small piece of fruit, half a cup of quinoa or some other moderately starchy carb and a serving of protein. Use your food app to make sure you're getting the correct amount of carbs and to keep track of your carb budget.

Please do not eat sweets and please do not *add* fat to this meal with the carbs. We do not want high fat and high carb together. 20-40 grams of protein and 10-15 grams of carbs or 20-40 grams of protein, fat (i.e. butter, avocado, olive oil, nuts) and non-starchy vegetables. You do not have to have the carbs after the workout if you can get by without them and want to be more aggressive with your weight loss. However, if you are feeling very fatigued or hungry after your workout, then a small serving of carbs may keep you from giving in to a stronger craving later in the day and make sure you are ready for tomorrow's workout.

Testimonial from Remote Coaching Client:

I remember THE DAY…when I was exhausted from trying to figure out "WHY AM I NOT LOSING WEIGHT…I AM TRYING!" Who knew I was saying that out loud to the RIGHT PERSON…My sweet friend, Danielle said "Call Zane (her husband) he can help!" Best advice ever…Zane was not judgmental and I could tell from the first

conversation he was going to HELP ME! We talked about my eating, skipping meals, exercising and what I was missing. I'm a former Chef…so dieting just wasn't the answer. Talking with Zane helped me see that I needed to TWEAK my mindset…and it was about committing to the lifestyle of healthy living! So grateful for the coaching…I have lost 35 pounds and maintained the weight loss. I've never been a more confident ANDRIKA!!!

-Andrika Langham, Knoxville, TN

CHAPTER 9

SLEEP TIGHT

You have to speak words of continuous encouragement in order to achieve whatever goals you've set for yourself.
-Anquanette Gaspard

Sleep plays an important role in the regulation of the hormones affecting blood sugar regulation and hunger.[10] A lack of sleep has been shown to cause an increase in insulin resistance, meaning that less fuel is going to the muscles and more is being stored as fat. It can also cause a decrease in the hormone leptin which causes us to feel satisfied and an increase in the hormone ghrelin which causes us to feel hungry. Elevated levels of the stress hormone cortisol which can add to fat storage, also result from a lack of sleep. Many studies show these effects on our hormones taking place in as little as two to five days of insufficient sleep.

The Sleep Heart Health Study found that sleep durations of six hours or less or nine hours or more were associated with an increased prevalence of Type 2 Diabetes when compared to seven to eight hours of sleep. Several studies on this subject have shown that a lack or disturbance of sleep can have negative effects on insulin sensitivity and appetite and an increased risk of obesity, Type 2 Diabetes and non-alcoholic fatty liver disease.[11]

I made sure when I felt the need to eat something crunchy I ate nuts instead and stayed away from the carbs.
-Jennifer Hudson, Singer, Actress

Consuming alcohol in the evening can have a disruptive effect on sleep. I have found this to be more common with my clients over the age of 40. While alcohol is a depressant and can "take the edge off" helping us to relax and even get to sleep, many people find themselves waking up with their heart pounding in the middle of the night. When drinking alcohol our bodies respond by releasing adrenaline to counter the depressant effects. Once the alcohol has been processed our bodies will reduce the adrenaline being released but for many people their adrenaline level is not reduced quickly enough and they are suddenly wide awake when they should be in a deep sleep.

Another sleep disturbing factor is over exposure to ultraviolet light from the screens of our phones, computers and other devices. The blue light from these devices has a delaying effect on our circadian rhythm, our body's internal clock, causing a longer time to get to sleep, reduced REM sleep and a longer time to wake up in the morning.[12] It has also been shown to decrease the production of the hormones serotonin and melatonin which our bodies use for sleep.[13]

The general recommendation is to reduce exposure to blue light at least two hours before bedtime.[14] Ideally this means getting off of the devices altogether two hours before going to bed but there are a couple of things you can do to help reduce blue light exposure while looking at a screen. You can use an ultraviolet reducing app on your device like flux that gradually reduces the amount of blue light being used on the screen as you get closer to bedtime. You can also wear blue light filtering glasses while using a screen in the evening.

There are many factors that can negatively affect the body's production of melatonin so taking a melatonin supplement may be helpful for you. Make sure the room is as dark as possible so remove nightlights, use thick drapes and cover or remove any devices emitting light, especially blue light. The recommended room temperature for sleep is between 60 and 67 degrees Fahrenheit or between 15 and 20 degrees Celsius. Make it your sleep cave.

Testimonial from *Extreme Weight Loss* TV Show:

I spent a lot of time working with Zane during season 4 of ABC's Extreme Weight Loss. His knowledge and guidance helped me not only lose the weight, but also to tone up and hit my end goal for the finale. I recommend Zane to anybody who is ready to make a change!

-Jayce Hein, Nashville, TN

CHAPTER 10

HOW DO I KNOW HOW MUCH FAT OR CARBOHYDRATE I AM EATING?

No matter the number of times you fail you must be determined to succeed. You must not lose hope. Don't stop in your storm.

-Tony Narams

Making the transition from high carb to high fat is a paradigm shift for most people. To do it successfully you will need to know how much fat and carbohydrate you're eating. I strongly suggest using a food app, like *MyFitnessPal*, or another app that allows you to see the macronutrient ratio of fat, carbs and protein you have eaten and allows you to change the goals for each of those.

In general, your goal ratios should look like this: 55-70% fat, 20-25% protein and 5-15% carbohydrate. If your goal is weight loss, you will have to adjust your carb intake to the point that allows you to lose weight consistently. For some, 15% from carbohydrates will work and others will need to go lower. Managing your carb budget is the most important factor in your weight loss. In my experience, many people find their carb goal for weight loss somewhere between 80 and 150 grams of net carbs per day. The net carbs is the total carbohydrate intake minus the fiber.

I love eating sushi and eating raw and clean - no pasta and bread. Low carbs is what works for me.

-Chrissy Teigen, Model, Actress

The carbs you will have to reduce are the starchy and sugary kind like potatoes, fruit, beans, grains and sweets. You will want to eat a lot of non-starchy vegetables which don't add much "carb" to your carb count. Most of the carbs in these veggies are fiber which cannot be burned for fuel and will not inhibit fat burning but they do feed your biome. After some practice, you will learn how to gauge your servings of sugar and starch. In general, the majority of your plate, and what you eat in a day, should be non-starchy vegetables.

15

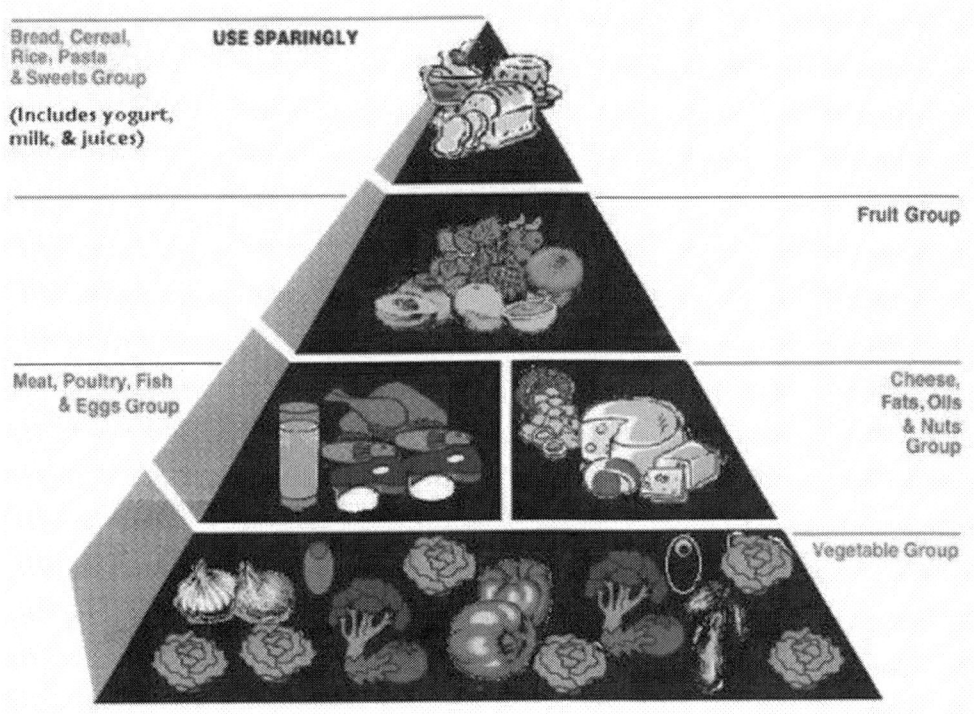

The differences between these two food pyramids are obvious. The first one is the USDA pyramid recommended by health authorities for decades now. 6-11 servings of grains? It is no wonder that 60% of the US population is overweight or obese. There are even more carbs to eat as you go up the pyramid, like fruit and legumes. On the second pyramid, that same "grain" category is moved to the smallest serving and vegetables make up the largest group. Obviously fat has a much larger place on the new pyramid too.

From the Food Comes First 30 Day Weight Loss Facebook Group:

My favorite thing about this program is that I haven't felt hungry or deprived once! This is the FIRST 'diet' I can actually see turning into a lifestyle change. It's so doable, and the results are amazing! 11 pounds in 30 days eating food I actually enjoy? Why am I just now doing this? Thanks, Zane, for your incredible coaching, encouragement and accountability!

-Chance S., Franklin, TN

CHAPTER 11

LET'S GO SHOPPING!

Don't make a habit out of choosing what feels good over what's actually good for you.

– Eric Thomas

Your Shopping List:

These foods will make up the majority of your diet.

Vegetables: broccoli, asparagus, Brussels sprouts, green beans, garlic, onions, kale, spinach, dark leafy greens, artichokes, bok choy, cauliflower, mushrooms (yes, they're technically a fungus), lettuces, cabbage, sprouts and other non-starchy veggies. You may eat an unlimited amount of these. Fill up on them.

Proteins: whole eggs (yes, eat the yolks), beef (ideally grass fed), chicken and other poultry (ideally free range), wild caught fish (not farm raised), wild game, pork, shellfish

Fats: coconut oil, olive oil, butter, ghee, avocado, avocado oil, tree nuts, unsweetened nut butters, unsweetened almond or coconut milk, olives, seeds, cheese in small amounts, beef tallow, duck fat

Low Sugar Fruit: bell pepper, cucumber, tomatoes, squash of all kinds including zucchini, eggplant, lemon, lime. Use these foods to help fill you up, replace starchy carbs and provide slow burning energy.

Fermented Food: These are great for feeding the biome: kombucha, unpasteurized kimchi and sauerkraut, fermented meat and eggs, pickled fruit and veggies (in brine, not vinegar) like olives or peppers.

Prebiotic Foods: The fiber of certain foods are known as prebiotic and are preferred food for the healthy bacteria in our biome. Including these foods in your diet is highly recommended. These are the most common: raw Jerusalem artichoke, raw dandelion greens, raw garlic, raw or cooked onions, acacia gum, raw chicory root, raw asparagus and raw leek.

Foods to Limit: The following foods are eaten less frequently, as in a small portion each day or maybe 2-3 times a week, for example after a workout or as the carb portion of the evening meal.

Dairy: With milk, cream and half and half just use a little in coffee or for cooking if you need to. Kefir (preferable because it's fermented) and unsweetened plain Greek yogurt are good snack options.

Legumes: beans, peas, other legumes. Your portion size is 15g of net carb.

Whole fruit: berries, citrus, apples, peaches, pears, nectarines, melons, etc. Berries are the lowest glycemic and make a great dessert. Aim for a portion size of approximately 15g of net carb. This will be different for each fruit.

Grains without gluten: quinoa, rice (wild, brown, white), amaranth, corn, oats, buckwheat (not wheat). Your portion size is 15g of net carb.

Dark chocolate: 75% cocoa or higher, just a couple squares as a dessert. The higher the percentage, the lower the sugar and higher the antioxidants.

You may have a dessert after dinner if you haven't had a starch serving, i.e. berries or dark chocolate.

No calorie sweeteners: sweeteners like Stevia or sugar alcohols will still elevate insulin because they taste sweet and we are trying to avoid this whenever possible. If you are using these at the same time you are eating other food then the impact will not be as significant. Using them while fasting is counterproductive since one of the primary goals of fasting is to reduce insulin levels. If you are using it in your coffee or tea as a breakfast substitute then I recommend waiting until consistent weight loss has begun and to remove it if weight loss stalls. Avoid using it between meals because we want insulin levels to remain low during this time.

Supplements: I recommend taking a probiotic supplement with at least 30 billion units and 10 different strains at least 30 minutes before your first meal, or any meal if you forget.

Drinking coffee when you take the supplement could limit its effectiveness so don't drink coffee or other acidic drinks within 30 minutes of taking your probiotic.

Turmeric is a great natural anti-inflammatory. The recommended amount is at least 600mg a day.

Omega 3 fatty acids are another natural anti-inflammatory and we need them to balance out the Omega 6 fatty acids so prevalent in our diet. Aim for at least 1000mg a day and ideally

1000mg of DHA. EPA's will usually be included but you are after as much DHA as possible.

Take a multivitamin and mineral supplement of your choice. We can't possibly get all of the nutrients we need from our food.

Taking a prebiotic fiber supplement is a great way to feed your biome. Make sure it is labeled a prebiotic fiber.

Things to avoid:

Alcohol: 2-3 servings per week of wine or hard alcohol (straight or with a sugar free mixer like seltzer water). No beer. Alcohol is not your friend when it comes to losing weight so if you can abstain, that's better. Beer is one of the worst things you can drink when trying to lose weight. **No beer**.

Of all alcoholic drinks, wine is the least harmful to the biome because it is fermented and contains antioxidants, however, too much alcohol of any kind will harm the bacteria in your gut, act as a depressant to your whole system and limit weight loss.

No juice of ANY kind, sugar sweetened tea or coffee, sodas with sugar, smoothies, energy drinks with sugar....you get it. **No drinks with sugar**. You don't want to drink artificially sweetened drinks either. The taste, and even the smell, of something sweet causes a small release of insulin. We are trying to decrease insulin resistance and increase insulin sensitivity so frequent releases of insulin throughout your day, even from a no calorie drink like a diet soda, will not help. There is enough insulin activity from eating.

Grains containing gluten, primarily wheat, should be avoided because of their inflammatory effect on the gut, and our whole system in general, and because they raise blood sugar more than many other foods. Grains with gluten include wheat (or the wheat family like spelt, durum, farro, bulgar) rye, barley, triticale. Oats do not include gluten naturally but they are often processed in plants with wheat products so they may contain gluten from their processing. Please stick to the grains listed in "grains without gluten". This means that breakfast cereals, pasta, bread, couscous, crackers, many trail mixes and granola are not on your food list, no matter how healthy the packaging looks.

Avoid soy whenever possible. Soy is a phyto-estrogen which encourages fat storage and can create imbalances in your hormones. I realize that occasionally you may eat some form of processed food like a bar or bottled salad dressing containing soy because it is easy to overlook. You'll have to read labels, even on "healthy" food, because it's in more foods than you realize.

No carbs. No dairy. No refined sugar. [It's] eating real foods. It's honestly high-fat, high-protein. I think that we've been brainwashed to think that fat is bad, but really, it's what going to make you feel fuller longer. And your body can burn it and use it as fuel.

-Vanessa Hudgens, Actress

CHAPTER 12

THE MEAL PLAN

It is important to surround yourself with people who lift you up, encourage you, share your vision and inspire you.

-Les Brown

If you are taking insulin or some other drug to control your blood sugar please check with your doctor before starting your new eating plan. This is important because adjustments to your prescriptions may be required as insulin sensitivity improves. Do not do this yourself. If this is your situation, keep your doctor involved and informed.

On this plan, there are breakfasts, lunches, dinners and optional snacks but that doesn't mean you need to eat all of those every day. As a rule, if you're not hungry, don't eat. I've included them for variety and flexibility, not as a set number of meals you need to eat. Our culture eats too much and too often which inhibits fat burning. Time between meals allows our blood sugar to level out and insulin to drop so we can tap into our fat stores. If you can be satisfied with three meals a day then you don't need a snack. This should be your goal. Snacking between meals or grazing will inhibit weight loss.

If you're practicing intermittent fasting in the form of time restricted eating to 8 hours a day with a meal at midday, an afternoon snack and an evening meal while getting adequate calories, that's fantastic. Don't eat more or more often than you need to, especially while in weight loss mode. As a rule, you should eat all of your meals within 12 hours or less every day to allow for at least 12 hours during which you are unfed and insulin is not needed. If you eat breakfast at 7:00 am then you should finish your last meal or snack before 7:00 pm. If dinner is the most important meal on your schedule to be with family, etc. then start your meals in relation to your dinner time and delay your first meal as needed to compress your eating schedule.

If you're used to grazing all day or eating 5-6 times a day then you can start by transitioning to the three meals and a snack schedule if you find that only eating three meals a day is too big of a jump at first. Stick to whole foods and stay away from processed snack foods, even if they're labeled "low carb" or "keto friendly". Those items can sometimes be helpful in an emergency but should not be part of your regular diet.

I have included protein shakes in the breakfast and snack options as an alternative for when time is tight or to fit your eating schedule when healthy food options aren't available. For example, if you're trying to transition to eating breakfast later in the morning but eating a breakfast packed from home isn't an option then a shake with whey, greens and some healthy fats can help you work your way to breaking the fast with a full meal at lunch. Notice that pre-made shakes are not included. This is because most of the protein shakes in the stores include ingredients you don't want to eat such as added sugars, soy protein or preservatives. My recommendation is to find a grass fed, unsweetened whey protein and make your own shake like what I've listed.

Since the goal is to only eat three meals a day, or possibly two meals and a snack, you want those to be made up of real, whole, unprocessed foods that still have their nutrients and fiber intact.

Replace the homemade shake with a whole food meal as soon as possible. Whole food meals like what I've listed will take longer to digest, have less of an impact on insulin and give you more satiety.

Be wary of foods at restaurants that may sound like they are healthy or low carb because those foods often contain ingredients like extra sugar and starch that you don't realize. Restaurants and food producers are in the business of selling food, not helping people lose weight. They will add ingredients to food, like sugar or manmade sodium additives, to add flavor and make it more enjoyable so you will want to eat more of it. Items like soup or typically grain based foods that are labeled "gluten free" are good examples of this. The nutritional information of the food at most popular restaurants is available online and can be found with a quick search on your smart phone, so be on the offensive.

Good Morning! You are welcome to have coffee, tea or water. Just don't use sugar or any other sweetener like honey, turbinado or coconut sugar.

You can add fat like a tablespoon of butter and/or coconut oil. 2 oz. of heavy cream or half and half can also be used.

You can add Stevia as a sweetener after you have adjusted to a low carb diet and weight loss has begun, however if the weight loss stalls, eliminate it. You can choose to make this your only breakfast to put more of a demand on fat burning.

Breakfast: If you work out (resistance training) in the morning, after your workout, you can have a whey protein shake, 20-40g of protein, with water or 1 cup of unsweetened almond milk (unsweetened will be clearly marked) and a cup of berries. This is a great recovery meal for whenever you work out. You want 20-40g of protein and approximately 15g of carbohydrate. You can also have the shake without berries and eat a grapefruit, orange, peach, nectarine or half of a large (or one small) apple of the same serving amount. As an alternative, you can eat 3-5 eggs or another protein source providing 20-40g of protein with a serving of fruit equaling about 15g of carbohydrate that isn't fiber if you do not want a shake. For example, if your fruit serving has 19g of total carb and 3g of fiber that leaves 16g of carb that is not fiber. You can use a food app such as *MyFitnessPal* or Google to determine the net carb of any food.

If you do not work out in the morning, you are welcome to skip breakfast and allow your body to rely primarily on fat stores through the morning until your first meal. The coffee or tea as described before is a good alternative.

If you eat breakfast on a non-workout day, you can have the whey shake without fruit, 3-5 eggs or other protein source. Instead of fruit, you can have raw, steamed or sautéed fibrous (non-starchy) veggies, i.e. green salad, asparagus, Brussels sprouts, broccoli, kale, etc. Salad dressing should be olive oil with vinegar, salt and pepper. Cook the eggs and veggies in coconut oil, butter or ghee. You can also add butter to the veggies, especially if you steam them. Try adding a handful of raw spinach to your whey shake to get some added greens. You will not taste the spinach but make sure you blend it well.

Lunch: You should eat about 6-8 oz. of your choice of protein: fish, beef, chicken, pork, eggs (3-5), etc. and a salad of veggies only using a dressing with no added sugar. Ideally make your own dressing with vinegar, olive oil, salt and pepper.

You can add steamed or sautéed veggies like broccoli, asparagus, cauliflower, Brussels sprouts, kale, green beans with butter and/or 1-2 oz. of cheese for some fat.

You may also add foods from the low sugar fruit list like squash, bell peppers, etc.

Afternoon Snack: (to replace a meal) You can choose from cheese, almonds, walnuts and any non-starchy veggies. Coffee or tea, black or with cream and stevia is fine- your choice. A protein like a whey shake with or without fruit, or some kind of meat or eggs is also fine. Only add fruit if you did not have it in your shake earlier in the day.

One piece or cup of fruit if you have not had any yet that day: citrus, apple, berries as noted above. 15g of net carb after deducting fiber. Limit fruit to 2-3 times a week.

Afternoon Workout: If you work out in the afternoon/evening, do it before dinner and allow at least 2 hours from your last meal or snack before your workout. This is to allow your blood sugar to come back down and improve fat burning.

Dinner: You should eat 6-8 oz. of a protein as listed above and a salad with no sugar in the dressing, but added cheese is fine. You should also have steamed or sautéed veggies with butter and/or cheese. Foods from the low sugar fruit list are also great to help fill you up at dinner. At this meal you can have a half serving of a starch such as the listed non-gluten grains, peas, beans, 1 corn tortilla, etc. equaling 15-20 grams or half a cup.

I know this will be a big reduction of starchy carbs for many of you. If you feel you need a transition period to work your way to this, start by having a full serving of your starchy carb at dinner equaling 30-40 grams. You can use a food app. or Google to determine the correct serving size of your carb choice.
If you are going to eat a dessert then skip the starch serving at dinner.

If you are ready for a more aggressive approach, you can substitute half a cup of nuts like almonds, cashews or walnuts for your carb serving on alternate days. Eat them as an after dinner snack but not with a dessert. If your weight loss is stuck, dessert should be the first to go.

Dessert: My suggested dessert is a cup of berries with cream. You can use heavy whipping cream and whip it up- just do not add sugar or honey. You can add a packet of stevia to the cream if necessary.

A couple squares of dark chocolate of 75% cocoa or higher is also an option. The higher the cocoa percentage, the lower the sugar.

Cheat Meal: As an option, you can have one cheat meal per week. If you can go without it then please do. Some people find that a cheat meal triggers cravings or causes them to gain 2-3 lbs. which they have to spend the following day or two trying to lose. If you are in weight loss mode and a cheat meal appears to slow your progress then you may want to wait until you are in maintenance mode to include it in your week. Remember, it is one cheat meal, not an entire cheat day.

If at some point your weight loss gets stuck or plateaus, do not get frustrated. Weight loss often comes in stair steps of progress and the scale may not always reveal it. Take measurements of the areas that seem to carry the most fat like your waist, hips, thighs, arms- wherever those places are on your body- and check them periodically. If you are losing size, you are moving in the right direction, whether the scale is moving much or not.

Starchy carbohydrates are energy foods so the more you eat, the less your body has to rely on fat stores for fuel. Look for hidden sugars in your food and drinks. You may need to cut back on sweet fruit or have your carb portion on fewer days until weight

loss begins again. You could also try substituting half a cup of nuts for your starchy carbs as I mentioned above.

A 2017 low carbohydrate diet study conducted at Indiana University and published in the journal JMIR Diabetes, involving 262 adults with Type II Diabetes, found that 87% of subjects were able to reduce or eliminate their need for medication to manage their disease. And this happened within a matter of weeks sometimes even days.

-Dr. David Harper, Associate professor of kinesiology at the University of the Fraser Valley, Visiting scientists at the B.C. Cancer Research Centre, Member of the scientific advisory board of the Institute for Personalized Therapeutic Nutrition

CHAPTER 13

LET'S EAT!

If you have made mistakes, there is always another chance for you. You may have a fresh start any moment you choose, for this thing we call 'failure' is not the falling down, but the staying down.

– Mary Pickford

I have included the following meals as examples to show just how well you can eat on a low carb plan and to stimulate your creative, culinary juices for preparing your own food. Try these meals for yourself and then make appropriate substitutions to fit your taste. Exchange protein for protein, fibrous vegetable for fibrous vegetable, fat for fat, etc. in the same serving sizes and create your own low carb favorites.

Meal Suggestions

Breakfast:
1. 3-4 scrambled eggs with sautéed onions, mushrooms, spinach. Use coconut oil or butter for cooking. Avocado on the side.

2. 3-4 fried eggs cooked with asparagus and/or Brussels sprouts in coconut oil or butter

3. 4-6 oz. of smoked salmon (lox) with 2 oz. of cheese and sliced avocado.

4. 3-4 hard-boiled eggs with steamed broccoli and/or cauliflower garnished with shredded cheese and/or butter.

5. Protein shake with unsweetened whey protein and unsweetened almond or coconut milk. Optionally you may add a tablespoon of unsweetened almond butter to the shake.

6. 3-4 fried eggs with sautéed greens (kale, spinach, collard) cooked in coconut oil or butter. Optionally add 2-3 oz. of feta cheese

7. 3-4 boiled eggs with asparagus and butter

8. Coffee or tea with butter, heavy cream or unsweetened coconut milk. Cinnamon optional

9. 3-4 egg omelet with mushrooms, spinach and grated parmesan.

10. 3 oz of steak, 2 fried eggs with sliced tomatoes

11. 4-6 oz of smoked salmon with sliced cucumber, tomato and 2 oz of cheese

12. 3-4 Scrambled eggs with sautéed spinach and sliced tomatoes

13. 3-4 egg frittata with spinach, bacon and shredded cheese

14. 4-6 oz of prosciutto with steamed or sautéed asparagus

15. 2 scrambled eggs with spinach and 3 oz leftover fish

16. 4 Deviled eggs with sliced avocado and tomato

17. 4-6 oz of leftover steak with sliced tomato

18. 2 Tablespoons of unsweetened almond butter with celery

19. 3 Egg muffins baked with cheese and crumbled bacon

20. Smoothie with ½ avocado, unsweetened coconut milk, unsweetened almond butter, 1 tbsp. unsweetened cocoa powder and ½ teaspoon cinnamon. Optional: stevia

21. Scramble with 3-4 eggs, ½ cup chopped zucchini, 1 chopped garlic clove

22. Iced latte with cooled black coffee or tea blended with ¼ cup unsweetened coconut milk, 1 teaspoon vanilla extract and ice. Optional: stevia

23. 3 poached eggs with steamed broccolini covered with butter

24. 3 oz of sausage with 2 fried eggs and sautéed spinach

25. Shake with unsweetened chocolate whey protein, unsweetened coconut milk, ¼ avocado, ½ cup raw spinach, tbsp. of unsweetened almond butter

26. Green smoothie with ½ avocado, 1 cup unsweetened coconut milk, 1 cup raw spinach, ½ chopped cucumber, 2 tbsp. fresh lemon juice or apple cider vinegar, water as needed

27. Shake with unsweetened vanilla whey protein, 1 cup unsweetened coconut milk, ½ cup chopped cucumber, 1 cup raw spinach, 1 cup blueberries, water as needed

28. Scramble with 3-4 eggs, 1 cup kale and ½ cup chopped tomato

29. 4-6 oz. of leftover fish sautéed with 1 cup spinach, served with ¼ avocado

30. Hot coffee blended with 1-2 tbsp. grass fed butter, 2 tsp. MCT oil, 1 tsp. turmeric. Optional: 1 tsp. cinnamon

Lunch:

1. 6 oz of pulled pork with a green salad and ½ cup of kimchi

2. 6 oz of sliced steak and ¼ avocado in a large green salad

3. 4 oz of cooked shrimp and 1 chopped avocado mixed with 2 tsp of lemon juice. Salt and pepper to taste. Optional: sugar free hot sauce, Sriracha sauce

4. 4 deviled eggs and 2 strips of bacon cut into 1 inch pieces in a large green salad with tomatoes

5. 1 bun-less burger (cheese optional) served in a large green salad with ¼ chopped avocado

6. 1 hamburger (cheese optional) served in a large lettuce leaf with sliced avocado and tomato

7. 6 oz of chicken salad served in a large green salad

8. 4 oz of smoked salmon, ½ cup full fat cream cheese and ½ chopped cucumber wrapped in rolled in nori sushi wraps

9. 4 oz of tuna salad and 2 hard-boiled eggs with sliced tomato and romaine leaves

10. 6 oz of meatballs in marinara sauce with sautéed ½ cup zucchini and a bell pepper

11. 1 6 oz. can of salmon mixed with avocado mayo and 2 tbsp. of fresh lemon juice, tossed in a large green salad with ¼ - ½ an avocado. Add olive oil as needed.

12. 1 6 oz. can of lump crab meat (optional: mix with 1-2 tsp of prepared horseradish) mixed in a large green salad with ¼ avocado and 2 tbsp. of fresh lemon juice. Add olive oil as needed.

13. 3-4 oz prosciutto served with a mix of 2 oz mozzarella balls, ½ cup chopped cherry tomatoes and ¼ chopped avocado in olive oil. Salt and pepper to taste.

14. Large Greek salad with 2-3 oz. of feta cheese, olives, bell pepper, tomato, red onion, cucumber and romaine lettuce in a dressing of olive oil and red wine vinegar. Salt and pepper to taste. Optional: chicken or fish can be added for more protein.

15. 6 oz. shredded chicken breast mixed with ½ chopped avocado in a large green salad with 2 tbsp. salsa with no sugar added and olive oil as needed. Optional: add shredded cheese and hot sauce

16. 1 grilled or baked chicken thigh with 1 cup or more of zucchini, steamed or sautéed in coconut oil

17. Cobb salad with 3 oz. of chopped ham, 3 sliced hard-boiled eggs, ½ sliced avocado in a large green salad dressed with olive oil and red wine vinegar. Salt and pepper to taste. Optional: add shredded cheese

18. 6 oz steak with 1 cup or more of steamed broccoli with melted butter

19. 6 oz pork chop with 1 cup or more of green beans with melted butter

20. Frittata with 3-4 eggs, zucchini, spinach and grated Romano cheese cooked in coconut oil or butter

21. Pan fry 6 oz. of chopped chicken breast, 1 cup broccoli, 1 cup raw spinach, 2 cloves of garlic and 1 chopped tomato cooked in coconut oil

22. 6 oz of chicken salad scooped into two halves of a raw bell pepper

23. 4 oz of chopped Italian sausage mixed with sautéed bell pepper, onion and tomatoes. 6-8 oz. of grilled chicken with a vegetable salad and steamed broccoli and/or cauliflower with butter and/or cheese

24. Beef or chicken fajitas with sautéed onions, peppers and tomatoes. Add avocado or guacamole and cheese. No tortillas or chips

25. Grilled fish with a vegetable salad and steamed or sautéed veggies like asparagus, Brussels sprouts or green beans topped with butter

26. Pork loin with unpasteurized sauerkraut and grilled or roasted zucchini, mushrooms, garlic and tomatoes

27. Taco-less taco salad with ground beef, shredded cheese, lettuce, tomato, red onion, sugar free salsa, bell peppers and avocado/guacamole. Dress with olive oil as needed. No chips or beans. If you don't like salsa, add red wine vinegar to olive oil for dressing.

28. Roasted chicken (white or dark meat) with cooked kale, collard greens and tomato. Side of grilled or sautéed squash.

29. Salmon in a salad of a variety of lettuces, red onion, tomato, feta cheese, pecans or walnuts, with oil and vinegar dressing. Side of steamed broccoli dressed with butter.

30. 6-8 oz. of grilled chicken with a vegetable salad and steamed broccoli and/or cauliflower with butter and/or cheese

Dinner:
1. Greek salad with 4-6 oz. chopped chicken breast, olives, bell pepper, tomato, cucumber, red onion, romaine lettuce and ½ cup of precooked chickpeas. Dress with olive oil and red wine vinegar.

2. 6 oz of ground beef mixed with 1 cup of spaghetti sauce served over 1 cup of spaghetti squash. Add a green salad dressed with olive oil and vinegar.

3. Stuffed bell peppers baked with ground beef, bell peppers, chopped tomato, shredded mozzarella cheese and minced garlic, drizzled with olive oil.

4. 6 oz. of chopped chicken breast stir fried in coconut oil with bok choy, broccoli and zucchini noodles served with 1 cup of riced cauliflower

5. 6 oz. of beef flank steak mixed with sautéed bell peppers and onion. Stir in ¼ chopped avocado and ½ cup tomatoes.

6. 6 oz. of shrimp pan fried in lemon and butter or ghee and served over 2 cups zucchini noodles. Add butter, lemon and salt as needed.

7. Beef strips topped with shredded cheese and pico de gallo served in romaine leaf "tacos".

8. Baked cod topped with avocado slices and pico de gallo served in romaine leaf "tacos".

9. 6 oz. of beef brisket served with Brussels sprouts sautéed in coconut oil and 2 cups of cauliflower rice. Add a green salad for more vegetable fiber.

10. 6 oz. of sliced chicken breast pan fried in coconut oil with asparagus and sliced cherry tomatoes then tossed in pesto sauce. Serve with a green salad dressed with olive oil and vinegar.

11. 6 oz. chicken breast, ½ cup of cashews and bok choy sautéed in coconut oil. Then simmered in ½ cup of full fat coconut milk. Optional: Serve with 1 cup of shirataki noodles.

12. 6 oz. of chopped chicken breast, fresh garlic and oregano sautéed in coconut oil or butter. Serve with 8 oz. of shirataki noodles mixed with a sauce of 2 tbsp. melted butter and the juice of 1 lemon.

13. 6 oz. of roasted leg of lamb served with sautéed asparagus, ½ cup quinoa and a green salad.

14. 6 oz. of sliced lamb and 2 tbsp. of hummus tossed in a large salad with olives, cucumbers, tomatoes, red onion, baby spinach leaves and romaine lettuce, dressed with olive oil and red wine vinegar. Optional: add ½ cup feta cheese.

15. 6 oz. of baked cod served with 2 cups of riced cauliflower and a large green salad dressed with olive oil and red wine vinegar.

16. A large salad for 2: sauté 1lb. of shrimp in ghee or coconut oil. Toss in a mix of 1-2 cups of cucumber, ½ cup red onion, 1 cup bell pepper and 2 chopped avocados. Dress with a mix of 4 tbsp. olive oil and 2 tbsp. lemon juice.

17. 6 oz. of sliced flank steak stir fried in coconut oil with ½ cup zucchini noodles, ½ cup broccoli florets and a chopped bunch of baby bok choy. Mix in 2 tbsp. coconut aminos for the soy sauce effect but without the soy. Serve as is or with a cup of riced cauliflower.

18. 6 oz. of beef pot roast cooked in the crockpot served with 1-2 cups of Brussels sprouts sautéed in coconut oil and a green salad dressed with olive oil and red wine vinegar.

19. 6 oz. of sliced beef sautéed in coconut oil with 2 cups of cabbage or fresh coleslaw mix and served with 1 cup shirataki noodles

20. Italian style meatballs in marinara sauce served on 2 cups zucchini noodles. Add a large green salad dressed with olive oil and red wine vinegar.

21. 6 oz. seared ahi tuna steak served with 8-10 asparagus spears sautéed in coconut oil and a green salad. Optional: Add 1 cup of riced cauliflower

22. 1 cup of bean-less chili with ground beef, bell peppers, onion and chopped tomato served on 1 cup of cauliflower rice.

23. 6 oz of pulled pork, ½ chopped or mashed avocado and 2 tbsp. sour cream served in 2 romaine leaf tacos. Use hot sauce as desired.

24. Crockpot pork roast with a green salad, green beans cooked in coconut oil and an optional half cup of quinoa.

25. Taco-less taco salad with ground beef or shredded chicken, shredded cheese, lettuce, tomato, red onion, sugar free salsa, avocado/guacamole and a half cup of pinto or black beans (no sugar added to beans)

26. Grilled salmon in a salad of a variety of lettuces, strawberries, walnuts, feta cheese with an olive oil and vinegar dressing. Asparagus sautéed in coconut oil. Optional half cup of brown rice.

27. Grilled steak with Brussels sprouts, mushrooms and garlic sautéed in butter and coconut oil. Optional glass of red wine. Optional dessert of 2-3 squares of chocolate containing 75% or more cocoa and half a cup of cashews or other tree nut.

28. Grass fed beef burgers with cheese wrapped in a romaine lettuce leaf or on a salad of lettuce and tomato, with grilled zucchini, yellow squash and eggplant.

29. Grilled or baked cod with kimchi, steamed broccoli or cauliflower dressed with butter and shredded cheese. Optional half cup of wild rice.

30. Grilled chicken (white or dark meat) with a Greek salad and sautéed zucchini, tomatoes and garlic. Optional dessert: Cup of whipped heavy whipping cream, unsweetened, or sweetened with stevia, on top of a cup of berries.

Snacks:

1. 1 can of sardines with ½ cup of olives

2. Celery stalks with 2 tbsp. of unsweetened almond butter

3. 3-4 oz. of beef jerky

4. Green salad mixed with 2 tbsp. of hummus. Dress with olive oil and red wine vinegar as needed.

5. 1-2 sticks of mozzarella string cheese

6. 3 slices of bacon with 1 sliced tomato

7. Celery stalks with 2 tbsp. duck liver pate

8. 3 oz. of chicken salad on celery or rolled into a romaine lettuce leaf

9. 2 oz. of cheese and ½ cup of olives

10. 3 oz. of canned salmon mixed with 1 tbsp. avocado mayo eaten with sliced cucumber chips.

11. 3 oz. of prosciutto with avocado slices

12. 2-3 deviled eggs

13. ¼ cup of sunflower seeds (no shell)

14. ¼ cup raspberries and/or blackberries

15. ½ cup of coffee with ½ cup of unsweetened almond or coconut milk. Add 1 packet stevia and 1 tsp of vanilla extract if desired. Can use 2-4 oz. of heavy cream in place of nut milk.

16. ½ cup of hummus with sliced bell peppers

17. 1 medium or 6-8 baby raw carrots with ½ cup hummus

18. 3-4 oz. sliced turkey or roast beef and cheese rolled together

19. 1 cup cherry tomatoes with ½ cup mozzarella cheese balls

20. 1 cup of bone broth

21. 1 cup of cold black or green tea blended with 1 cup unsweetened coconut milk and 1 packet stevia

22. 3 oz. of chevre or goat cheese with sliced cucumber

23. 1 can of smoked oysters with 1 sliced tomato

24. 2 tbsp. olive tapenade with celery stalks

25. A quarter to half of a cup of macadamia nuts, almonds, walnuts, pistachios

26. Raw veggies or low sugar fruit like bell peppers, cucumbers, tomatoes dipped in guacamole or with 2-3 oz. of cheese

27. One piece or serving of sweet fruit (apple, peach, grapefruit, berries) equaling approx. 15g of net carb if no fruit was previously eaten that day, or mixed in your shake. While losing weight, limit sweet fruit to a few times a week.

28. 1-2 hard-boiled eggs with tomatoes and bell pepper, or sliced and tossed in a green salad.

29. A protein shake with whey protein and unsweetened almond or coconut milk. Make sure the whey protein has at least 20g of protein and less than 5g of carb per serving. Look for whey protein sweetened with stevia rather than sugar.

30. The **F- Bomb**: half of an avocado mashed with a fork, mix in a tablespoon of olive oil and add salt, pepper and any other sugar free seasonings to zest it up like chili powder, red pepper, minced garlic, etc. (F=fat)

CHAPTER 14

TIME TO GET MOVING

Why should you continue going after your dreams? Because seeing the look on the faces of the people who said you couldn't... will be priceless.

– Kevin Ngo

Resistance Training Exercise Suggestions
This is in no way an exhaustive list or the only way I think you should work out. These are suggestions that I have found to be effective, time saving workouts. Please check my YouTube channel for examples of many of the exercises listed on the following chart.

▶ **Youtube.com/c/ZaneGriggs**

Full Body Circuits

3 Exercise:	Lower body, Upper body, Core
4 Exercise:	Lower body, Upper body Push, Core, Upper body Pull

2 Day Split

Day 1:	Lower body, Core
Day 2:	Upper body Push and Pull

Basic Exercise List

Upper body Push	chest press, push-ups, shoulder press, elevated or knee push-ups, triceps extension
Upper body Pull	rows, pulldowns, pull-ups, assisted pull-ups, reverse fly, biceps curl
Core	plank, side plank, leg lift, reverse crunch, seated tube twist, superman
Lower body	squat, deadlift, walking lunge, single leg squat, reverse lunge, side lunge, forward lunge, hip thrusters, hip bridges, single leg hip bridges, leg curl on ball, Romanian deadlift, clamshell with loop band

CHAPTER 15

PUT THE PLAN AND THE PLANNER TO WORK

The difficulty, the ordeal, is to start.

–Zane Grey

You have the plan. Now, it's up to you to put it to work. Fill your fridge with the food you're going to be eating and get the food that will hinder your progress out of sight....or just out. Put encouraging words, images and goals where you will see them throughout the day. If you have a strong reason for losing weight like a wedding, a particular activity or just being able to keep up with your kids, put a reminder of that reason out where you can see it to motivate you to stay on course.

Using the Planner

I have designed a one year daily planner to be a helpful tool for you to manage and track your progress with this plan. There is a one month example of the daily planner at the end of this book. If you feel like this would help you with changing habits and continuing with a low carb lifestyle then you can order one at Lulu.com or download it for free from my website, zanegriggs.com.

Let's be honest, YOU are the real planner here but it was my intention to create a simple, organized, interactive tool for both personal accountability *and* recognition. If you can check a box, you can follow this plan.... and doesn't it feel good to check something off of your list?

There are options in the planner for variation in your day because not every day is the same and *stuff* happens. You will see "post workout carbs" in both the breakfast and lunch boxes depending on when or if you work out that day. Fruit is listed in the snack section so that as you are limiting fruit intake you can look back and see how many times you have had it that week. Dinner lists carbs, fat and dessert for you to choose one, not all three. Vegetables are in every meal box to help you to remember to include them as often as possible and to be able to look back and see how that habit has improved.

The same is true for the exercise and activity boxes. You will not do all of those every day but you will have a record of what you *have* done….which is less for you to remember. There are spaces to write in your particular exercise option like a yoga or boot camp class, a recreational sport with your friends or at the park with your kids and a space for floor exercises while watching your favorite show. Movement is a vital part of a healthy lifestyle and you have to get it in when you can.

There is even a box to check off how you feel that day or write one in. You are likely to check more than one feeling…but hopefully not all.

Changing habits, especially eating habits, is very difficult. You are going to have several temptations and moments of weakness along the way. Visual reminders are very helpful but at some point you are probably going to make a decision that takes you "off plan". Do not let that one decision derail your progress. Take a moment and think about why you allowed that short moment to be more important than your long term goals, then dust yourself off and get back on the plan. Forget all of the reasons you think you cannot do this and believe the one reason that you can. Make that reason bigger than anything that would get in the way of your success. Success is a choice, not a feeling. Decide to be successful, stick to your plan and you will reach your goal.

I would love to hear how you are doing on your low carb lifestyle so please reach out to me by:

zane@zanegriggs.com
zanesblog
zanegriggsfitness
www.zanegriggs.com

Below is a list of some of my favorite books regarding the benefits of a low carbohydrate diet and the misconceptions about dietary fat.

The Obesity Code by Jason Fung, M.D.

The Diabetes Code by Jason Fung, M.D.

Deep Nutrition by Catherine Shanahan, M.D.

Good Calories, Bad Calories by Gary Taubes

Why We Get Fat, And What To Do About It by Gary Taubes

Grain Brain by David Perlmutter, M.D.

Brain Maker by David Perlmutter, M.D.

The Cure For Heart Disease by Dwight Lundell, M.D. and Todd R. Nordstrom

The Great Cholesterol Myth by Jonny Bowden, Ph.D. and Stephen Sinatra, M.D.

References

1. Opinion piece in the Vancouver Sun written by Dr. David Harper, April, 2018
https://vancouversun.com/opinion/op-ed/opinion-new-canada-food-guide-why-we-must-get-it-right-this-time

2. American Journal of Clinical Nutrition, March 2010: Analysis of 21 studies covering over 247,000 patients fund that the "intake of saturated fat was not associated with an increased risk of CHD, stroke, or CVD."
https://academic.oup.com/ajcn/article/91/3/535/4597110

3. Journal of Internal Medicine, August, 2005: Malmo Diet and Cancer Study shows more than 30% of calories from total fat and more than 10% of calories from saturated fat shows no increased mortality. "Current dietary guidelines regarding fat intake" were "not supported".
https://onlinelibrary.wiley.com/doi/abs/10.1111/j.1365-2796.2005.01520.x

4. Nutrients, April 2018 published by the NIH: "Overall, recent intervention studies with eggs demonstrate that the additional dietary cholesterol does not negatively affect serum lipids, and in some cases, appears to improve lipoprotein particle profiles and HDL functionality."
https://www.ncbi.nlm.nih.gov/pmc/articles/PMC5946211/

5. Harvard Study on the F/B ratio in European children vs. Rural African Children published online August, 2010.
https://www.ncbi.nlm.nih.gov/pmc/articles/PMC2930426/

6. Harvard Study in JAMA, June, 2012: Effects of Dietary Composition on Energy Expenditure during Weight-Loss Maintenance
https://jamanetwork.com/journals/jama/fullarticle/1199154

7. Epidemiology Magazine, March, 1997: Framingham Study shows that butter consumption did not increase risk of heart disease but consumption of trans fats like margarine did increase the risk of chd.
https://journals.lww.com/epidem/Abstract/1997/03000/Margarine_Intake_and_Subsequent_Coronary_Heart.8.aspx

8. New York Times Article on Biggest Loser Participants, May, 2016.
https://www.nytimes.com/2016/05/02/health/biggest-loser-weight-loss.html

9. Science Direct: Autonomic Nervous System: Sympathetic and Parasympathetic Nervous Systems
https://www.sciencedirect.com/topics/medicine-and-dentistry/autonomic-nervous-system

10. PMC, June, 2009: Effects of sleep disturbance on insulin resistance, appetite and risk of type 2 diabetes.
https://www.ncbi.nlm.nih.gov/pmc/articles/PMC2697035/

11. American Journal of Physiology, November, 2018: Effects of sleep disturbance on the risk of non-alcoholic fatty liver disease and insulin resistance.
https://www.physiology.org/doi/abs/10.1152/ajpendo.00072.2018

12. Scientific American, September, 2015: Blue light exposure has a negative effect on the circadian rhythm.
https://www.scientificamerican.com/article/q-a-why-is-blue-light-before-bedtime-bad-for-sleep/

13. Pub. Med., January-April, 1999: Ultraviolet light exposure affects serotonin and melatonin production
https://www.ncbi.nlm.nih.gov/pubmed/10085464

14. Science News for Students, November, 2017: Eliminate screen time two hours before going to bed.
https://www.sciencenewsforstudents.org/article/evening-screen-time-can-sabotage-sleep

15. USDA food pyramid 1992
https://www.choosemyplate.gov/brief-history-usda-food-guides

16. Low carb food pyramid
http://www.theketogenicdiet.org/what-is-the-ketogenic-diet/

Daily Planner

In the following pages I have included a 31 day version of the daily planner to help you make the plan in this book a part of your daily life. The interactive planner allows you to check off your daily food and activity choices. If you can check a box, you can follow this plan.

If you find this helpful, you can purchase a spiral bound, one year planner at Lulu.com by searching my name or download a free PDF version at zanegriggs.com.

1 DAY

M T W T F S S

BREAKFAST
- ○ Skipped It
- ○ Coffee or Tea Only
- ○ Protein 20-40g
- ○ Post Workout Carbs
- ○ Vegetables
- ○ Fat

LUNCH
- ○ Protein 20-40g
- ○ Vegetables
- ○ Fat
- ○ Post Workout Carbs

NOTES
_____
_____
_____
_____

AFTERNOON SNACK
- ○ Protein 20-40g
- ○ Vegetables
- ○ Fat
- ○ Fruit

DINNER
- ○ Protein 20-40g
- ○ Vegetables
- ○ Carb Serving
- ○ Fat
- ○ Dessert

EXERCISE
- ○ Strength Training
- ○ Cardio
  _____
- ○ Other
  _____

ADDITIONAL ACTIVITIES
- ○ Brisk Walk
- ○ Recreational Activity
  _____
- ○ Took the Stairs
- ○ Yard Work
- ○ While Watching TV
  _____
- ○ Furthest Parking Spot
- ○ Other
  _____

HOW DO I FEEL?
- ○ Totally Awesome
- ○ Energetic
- ○ Motivated
- ○ Satisfied
- ○ Hungry
- ○ Moody
- ○ Lethargic
- ○ Stressed
- ○ Need Sleep
- ○ Other
  _____

2 DAY
M T W T F S S

BREAKFAST
- ○ Skipped It
- ○ Coffee or Tea Only
- ○ Protein 20-40g
- ○ Post Workout Carbs
- ○ Vegetables
- ○ Fat

AFTERNOON SNACK
- ○ Protein 20-40g
- ○ Vegetables
- ○ Fat
- ○ Fruit

DINNER
- ○ Protein 20-40g
- ○ Vegetables
- ○ Carb Serving
- ○ Fat
- ○ Dessert

ADDITIONAL ACTIVITIES
- ○ Brisk Walk
- ○ Recreational Activity

_____

- ○ Took the Stairs
- ○ Yard Work
- ○ While Watching TV

_____

- ○ Furthest Parking Spot
- ○ Other

_____

LUNCH
- ○ Protein 20-40g
- ○ Vegetables
- ○ Fat
- ○ Post Workout Carbs

EXERCISE
- ○ Strength Training
- ○ Cardio

_____

- ○ Other

_____

HOW DO I FEEL?
- ○ Totally Awesome
- ○ Energetic
- ○ Motivated
- ○ Satisfied
- ○ Hungry
- ○ Moody
- ○ Lethargic
- ○ Stressed
- ○ Need Sleep
- ○ Other

_____

NOTES
_____
_____
_____
_____

3 DAY

M T W T F S S

BREAKFAST
- ○ Skipped It
- ○ Coffee or Tea Only
- ○ Protein 20-40g
- ○ Post Workout Carbs
- ○ Vegetables
- ○ Fat

LUNCH
- ○ Protein 20-40g
- ○ Vegetables
- ○ Fat
- ○ Post Workout Carbs

AFTERNOON SNACK
- ○ Protein 20-40g
- ○ Vegetables
- ○ Fat
- ○ Fruit

DINNER
- ○ Protein 20-40g
- ○ Vegetables
- ○ Carb Serving
- ○ Fat
- ○ Dessert

EXERCISE
- ○ Strength Training
- ○ Cardio
  _____
- ○ Other
  _____

ADDITIONAL ACTIVITIES
- ○ Brisk Walk
- ○ Recreational Activity
  _____
- ○ Took the Stairs
- ○ Yard Work
- ○ While Watching TV
  _____
- ○ Furthest Parking Spot
- ○ Other
  _____

HOW DO I FEEL?
- ○ Totally Awesome
- ○ Energetic
- ○ Motivated
- ○ Satisfied
- ○ Hungry
- ○ Moody
- ○ Lethargic
- ○ Stressed
- ○ Need Sleep
- ○ Other
  _____

NOTES
_____
_____
_____
_____

DAY 4

M T W T F S S

BREAKFAST
- ○ Skipped It
- ○ Coffee or Tea Only
- ○ Protein 20-40g
- ○ Post Workout Carbs
- ○ Vegetables
- ○ Fat

LUNCH
- ○ Protein 20-40g
- ○ Vegetables
- ○ Fat
- ○ Post Workout Carbs

AFTERNOON SNACK
- ○ Protein 20-40g
- ○ Vegetables
- ○ Fat
- ○ Fruit

DINNER
- ○ Protein 20-40g
- ○ Vegetables
- ○ Carb Serving
- ○ Fat
- ○ Dessert

EXERCISE
- ○ Strength Training
- ○ Cardio
- _____
- ○ Other
- _____

ADDITIONAL ACTIVITIES
- ○ Brisk Walk
- ○ Recreational Activity
- _____
- ○ Took the Stairs
- ○ Yard Work
- ○ While Watching TV
- _____
- ○ Furthest Parking Spot
- ○ Other
- _____

HOW DO I FEEL?
- ○ Totally Awesome
- ○ Energetic
- ○ Motivated
- ○ Satisfied
- ○ Hungry
- ○ Moody
- ○ Lethargic
- ○ Stressed
- ○ Need Sleep
- ○ Other
- _____

NOTES
_____
_____
_____
_____

5 DAY

M T W T F S S

BREAKFAST
- ○ Skipped It
- ○ Coffee or Tea Only
- ○ Protein 20-40g
- ○ Post Workout Carbs
- ○ Vegetables
- ○ Fat

LUNCH
- ○ Protein 20-40g
- ○ Vegetables
- ○ Fat
- ○ Post Workout Carbs

NOTES
_____
_____
_____
_____

AFTERNOON SNACK
- ○ Protein 20-40g
- ○ Vegetables
- ○ Fat
- ○ Fruit

DINNER
- ○ Protein 20-40g
- ○ Vegetables
- ○ Carb Serving
- ○ Fat
- ○ Dessert

EXERCISE
- ○ Strength Training
- ○ Cardio
  _____
- ○ Other
  _____

ADDITIONAL ACTIVITIES
- ○ Brisk Walk
- ○ Recreational Activity
  _____
- ○ Took the Stairs
- ○ Yard Work
- ○ While Watching TV
  _____
- ○ Furthest Parking Spot
- ○ Other
  _____

HOW DO I FEEL?
- ○ Totally Awesome
- ○ Energetic
- ○ Motivated
- ○ Satisfied
- ○ Hungry
- ○ Moody
- ○ Lethargic
- ○ Stressed
- ○ Need Sleep
- ○ Other
  _____

6 DAY
M T W T F S S

BREAKFAST
- ○ Skipped It
- ○ Coffee or Tea Only
- ○ Protein 20-40g
- ○ Post Workout Carbs
- ○ Vegetables
- ○ Fat

LUNCH
- ○ Protein 20-40g
- ○ Vegetables
- ○ Fat
- ○ Post Workout Carbs

NOTES
_____
_____
_____
_____

AFTERNOON SNACK
- ○ Protein 20-40g
- ○ Vegetables
- ○ Fat
- ○ Fruit

DINNER
- ○ Protein 20-40g
- ○ Vegetables
- ○ Carb Serving
- ○ Fat
- ○ Dessert

EXERCISE
- ○ Strength Training
- ○ Cardio
  _____
- ○ Other
  _____

ADDITIONAL ACTIVITIES
- ○ Brisk Walk
- ○ Recreational Activity

_____
- ○ Took the Stairs
- ○ Yard Work
- ○ While Watching TV

_____
- ○ Furthest Parking Spot
- ○ Other

_____

HOW DO I FEEL?
- ○ Totally Awesome
- ○ Energetic
- ○ Motivated
- ○ Satisfied
- ○ Hungry
- ○ Moody
- ○ Lethargic
- ○ Stressed
- ○ Need Sleep
- ○ Other

_____

7 DAY

M T W T F S S

BREAKFAST
- ○ Skipped It
- ○ Coffee or Tea Only
- ○ Protein 20-40g
- ○ Post Workout Carbs
- ○ Vegetables
- ○ Fat

LUNCH
- ○ Protein 20-40g
- ○ Vegetables
- ○ Fat
- ○ Post Workout Carbs

AFTERNOON SNACK
- ○ Protein 20-40g
- ○ Vegetables
- ○ Fat
- ○ Fruit

DINNER
- ○ Protein 20-40g
- ○ Vegetables
- ○ Carb Serving
- ○ Fat
- ○ Dessert

EXERCISE
- ○ Strength Training
- ○ Cardio
- ○ Other _____

ADDITIONAL ACTIVITIES
- ○ Brisk Walk
- ○ Recreational Activity _____
- ○ Took the Stairs
- ○ Yard Work
- ○ While Watching TV _____
- ○ Furthest Parking Spot
- ○ Other _____

HOW DO I FEEL?
- ○ Totally Awesome
- ○ Energetic
- ○ Motivated
- ○ Satisfied
- ○ Hungry
- ○ Moody
- ○ Lethargic
- ○ Stressed
- ○ Need Sleep
- ○ Other _____

NOTES
_____
_____
_____
_____

8 DAY

M T W T F S S

BREAKFAST
- ○ Skipped It
- ○ Coffee or Tea Only
- ○ Protein 20-40g
- ○ Post Workout Carbs
- ○ Vegetables
- ○ Fat

LUNCH
- ○ Protein 20-40g
- ○ Vegetables
- ○ Fat
- ○ Post Workout Carbs

AFTERNOON SNACK
- ○ Protein 20-40g
- ○ Vegetables
- ○ Fat
- ○ Fruit

DINNER
- ○ Protein 20-40g
- ○ Vegetables
- ○ Carb Serving
- ○ Fat
- ○ Dessert

EXERCISE
- ○ Strength Training
- ○ Cardio
  _____
- ○ Other
  _____

ADDITIONAL ACTIVITIES
- ○ Brisk Walk
- ○ Recreational Activity
  _____
- ○ Took the Stairs
- ○ Yard Work
- ○ While Watching TV
  _____
- ○ Furthest Parking Spot
- ○ Other
  _____

HOW DO I FEEL?
- ○ Totally Awesome
- ○ Energetic
- ○ Motivated
- ○ Satisfied
- ○ Hungry
- ○ Moody
- ○ Lethargic
- ○ Stressed
- ○ Need Sleep
- ○ Other
  _____

NOTES
_____
_____
_____
_____

9 DAY
M T W T F S S

BREAKFAST
- ○ Skipped It
- ○ Coffee or Tea Only
- ○ Protein 20-40g
- ○ Post Workout Carbs
- ○ Vegetables
- ○ Fat

LUNCH
- ○ Protein 20-40g
- ○ Vegetables
- ○ Fat
- ○ Post Workout Carbs

AFTERNOON SNACK
- ○ Protein 20-40g
- ○ Vegetables
- ○ Fat
- ○ Fruit

DINNER
- ○ Protein 20-40g
- ○ Vegetables
- ○ Carb Serving
- ○ Fat
- ○ Dessert

EXERCISE
- ○ Strength Training
- ○ Cardio
- ○ Other _____

ADDITIONAL ACTIVITIES
- ○ Brisk Walk
- ○ Recreational Activity
- _____
- ○ Took the Stairs
- ○ Yard Work
- ○ While Watching TV
- _____
- ○ Furthest Parking Spot
- ○ Other
- _____

HOW DO I FEEL?
- ○ Totally Awesome
- ○ Energetic
- ○ Motivated
- ○ Satisfied
- ○ Hungry
- ○ Moody
- ○ Lethargic
- ○ Stressed
- ○ Need Sleep
- ○ Other
- _____

NOTES
_____
_____
_____
_____

10 DAY

M T W T F S S

BREAKFAST
- ○ Skipped It
- ○ Coffee or Tea Only
- ○ Protein 20-40g
- ○ Post Workout Carbs
- ○ Vegetables
- ○ Fat

LUNCH
- ○ Protein 20-40g
- ○ Vegetables
- ○ Fat
- ○ Post Workout Carbs

AFTERNOON SNACK
- ○ Protein 20-40g
- ○ Vegetables
- ○ Fat
- ○ Fruit

DINNER
- ○ Protein 20-40g
- ○ Vegetables
- ○ Carb Serving
- ○ Fat
- ○ Dessert

EXERCISE
- ○ Strength Training
- ○ Cardio
- ○ Other _____

ADDITIONAL ACTIVITIES
- ○ Brisk Walk
- ○ Recreational Activity
- _____
- ○ Took the Stairs
- ○ Yard Work
- ○ While Watching TV
- _____
- ○ Furthest Parking Spot
- ○ Other
- _____

HOW DO I FEEL?
- ○ Totally Awesome
- ○ Energetic
- ○ Motivated
- ○ Satisfied
- ○ Hungry
- ○ Moody
- ○ Lethargic
- ○ Stressed
- ○ Need Sleep
- ○ Other
- _____

NOTES
_____
_____
_____
_____

11 DAY

M T W T F S S

BREAKFAST
- ☐ Skipped It
- ☐ Coffee or Tea Only
- ☐ Protein 20-40g
- ☐ Post Workout Carbs
- ☐ Vegetables
- ☐ Fat

LUNCH
- ☐ Protein 20-40g
- ☐ Vegetables
- ☐ Fat
- ☐ Post Workout Carbs

AFTERNOON SNACK
- ☐ Protein 20-40g
- ☐ Vegetables
- ☐ Fat
- ☐ Fruit

DINNER
- ☐ Protein 20-40g
- ☐ Vegetables
- ☐ Carb Serving
- ☐ Fat
- ☐ Dessert

EXERCISE
- ☐ Strength Training
- ☐ Cardio
- ☐ Other _____

ADDITIONAL ACTIVITIES
- ☐ Brisk Walk
- ☐ Recreational Activity
_____
- ☐ Took the Stairs
- ☐ Yard Work
- ☐ While Watching TV
_____
- ☐ Furthest Parking Spot
- ☐ Other
_____

HOW DO I FEEL?
- ☐ Totally Awesome
- ☐ Energetic
- ☐ Motivated
- ☐ Satisfied
- ☐ Hungry
- ☐ Moody
- ☐ Lethargic
- ☐ Stressed
- ☐ Need Sleep
- ☐ Other
_____

NOTES
_____
_____
_____
_____

12 DAY

M T W T F S S

BREAKFAST
- ○ Skipped It
- ○ Coffee or Tea Only
- ○ Protein 20-40g
- ○ Post Workout Carbs
- ○ Vegetables
- ○ Fat

LUNCH
- ○ Protein 20-40g
- ○ Vegetables
- ○ Fat
- ○ Post Workout Carbs

AFTERNOON SNACK
- ○ Protein 20-40g
- ○ Vegetables
- ○ Fat
- ○ Fruit

DINNER
- ○ Protein 20-40g
- ○ Vegetables
- ○ Carb Serving
- ○ Fat
- ○ Dessert

EXERCISE
- ○ Strength Training
- ○ Cardio
- ○ Other _____

ADDITIONAL ACTIVITIES
- ○ Brisk Walk
- ○ Recreational Activity

_____

- ○ Took the Stairs
- ○ Yard Work
- ○ While Watching TV

_____

- ○ Furthest Parking Spot
- ○ Other

_____

HOW DO I FEEL?
- ○ Totally Awesome
- ○ Energetic
- ○ Motivated
- ○ Satisfied
- ○ Hungry
- ○ Moody
- ○ Lethargic
- ○ Stressed
- ○ Need Sleep
- ○ Other

_____

NOTES

_____
_____
_____
_____

13 DAY

M T W T F S S

BREAKFAST
- ○ Skipped It
- ○ Coffee or Tea Only
- ○ Protein 20-40g
- ○ Post Workout Carbs
- ○ Vegetables
- ○ Fat

AFTERNOON SNACK
- ○ Protein 20-40g
- ○ Vegetables
- ○ Fat
- ○ Fruit

DINNER
- ○ Protein 20-40g
- ○ Vegetables
- ○ Carb Serving
- ○ Fat
- ○ Dessert

ADDITIONAL ACTIVITIES
- ○ Brisk Walk
- ○ Recreational Activity
- _____
- ○ Took the Stairs
- ○ Yard Work
- ○ While Watching TV
- _____
- ○ Furthest Parking Spot
- ○ Other
- _____

LUNCH
- ○ Protein 20-40g
- ○ Vegetables
- ○ Fat
- ○ Post Workout Carbs

EXERCISE
- ○ Strength Training
- ○ Cardio
- _____
- ○ Other
- _____

HOW DO I FEEL?
- ○ Totally Awesome
- ○ Energetic
- ○ Motivated
- ○ Satisfied
- ○ Hungry
- ○ Moody
- ○ Lethargic
- ○ Stressed
- ○ Need Sleep
- ○ Other
- _____

NOTES
_____
_____
_____
_____

14 DAY

M T W T F S S

BREAKFAST
- ○ Skipped It
- ○ Coffee or Tea Only
- ○ Protein 20-40g
- ○ Post Workout Carbs
- ○ Vegetables
- ○ Fat

LUNCH
- ○ Protein 20-40g
- ○ Vegetables
- ○ Fat
- ○ Post Workout Carbs

NOTES

_____
_____
_____
_____

AFTERNOON SNACK
- ○ Protein 20-40g
- ○ Vegetables
- ○ Fat
- ○ Fruit

DINNER
- ○ Protein 20-40g
- ○ Vegetables
- ○ Carb Serving
- ○ Fat
- ○ Dessert

EXERCISE
- ○ Strength Training
- ○ Cardio
- _____
- ○ Other
- _____

ADDITIONAL ACTIVITIES
- ○ Brisk Walk
- ○ Recreational Activity
- _____
- ○ Took the Stairs
- ○ Yard Work
- ○ While Watching TV
- _____
- ○ Furthest Parking Spot
- ○ Other
- _____

HOW DO I FEEL?
- ○ Totally Awesome
- ○ Energetic
- ○ Motivated
- ○ Satisfied
- ○ Hungry
- ○ Moody
- ○ Lethargic
- ○ Stressed
- ○ Need Sleep
- ○ Other
- _____

15 DAY

M T W T F S S

BREAKFAST
- ○ Skipped It
- ○ Coffee or Tea Only
- ○ Protein 20-40g
- ○ Post Workout Carbs
- ○ Vegetables
- ○ Fat

LUNCH
- ○ Protein 20-40g
- ○ Vegetables
- ○ Fat
- ○ Post Workout Carbs

AFTERNOON SNACK
- ○ Protein 20-40g
- ○ Vegetables
- ○ Fat
- ○ Fruit

DINNER
- ○ Protein 20-40g
- ○ Vegetables
- ○ Carb Serving
- ○ Fat
- ○ Dessert

EXERCISE
- ○ Strength Training
- ○ Cardio
- ○ Other _____

ADDITIONAL ACTIVITIES
- ○ Brisk Walk
- ○ Recreational Activity _____
- ○ Took the Stairs
- ○ Yard Work
- ○ While Watching TV _____
- ○ Furthest Parking Spot
- ○ Other _____

HOW DO I FEEL?
- ○ Totally Awesome
- ○ Energetic
- ○ Motivated
- ○ Satisfied
- ○ Hungry
- ○ Moody
- ○ Lethargic
- ○ Stressed
- ○ Need Sleep
- ○ Other _____

NOTES
_____
_____
_____
_____

16 DAY

M T W T F S S

BREAKFAST
- ○ Skipped It
- ○ Coffee or Tea Only
- ○ Protein 20-40g
- ○ Post Workout Carbs
- ○ Vegetables
- ○ Fat

AFTERNOON SNACK
- ○ Protein 20-40g
- ○ Vegetables
- ○ Fat
- ○ Fruit

DINNER
- ○ Protein 20-40g
- ○ Vegetables
- ○ Carb Serving
- ○ Fat
- ○ Dessert

LUNCH
- ○ Protein 20-40g
- ○ Vegetables
- ○ Fat
- ○ Post Workout Carbs

EXERCISE
- ○ Strength Training
- ○ Cardio
- _____
- ○ Other
- _____

ADDITIONAL ACTIVITIES
- ○ Brisk Walk
- ○ Recreational Activity
- _____
- ○ Took the Stairs
- ○ Yard Work
- ○ While Watching TV
- _____
- ○ Furthest Parking Spot
- ○ Other
- _____

HOW DO I FEEL?
- ○ Totally Awesome
- ○ Energetic
- ○ Motivated
- ○ Satisfied
- ○ Hungry
- ○ Moody
- ○ Lethargic
- ○ Stressed
- ○ Need Sleep
- ○ Other
- _____

NOTES
_____
_____
_____
_____
_____

17 DAY

M T W T F S S

BREAKFAST
- ○ Skipped It
- ○ Coffee or Tea Only
- ○ Protein 20-40g
- ○ Post Workout Carbs
- ○ Vegetables
- ○ Fat

LUNCH
- ○ Protein 20-40g
- ○ Vegetables
- ○ Fat
- ○ Post Workout Carbs

AFTERNOON SNACK
- ○ Protein 20-40g
- ○ Vegetables
- ○ Fat
- ○ Fruit

DINNER
- ○ Protein 20-40g
- ○ Vegetables
- ○ Carb Serving
- ○ Fat
- ○ Dessert

EXERCISE
- ○ Strength Training
- ○ Cardio
- _____
- ○ Other
- _____

ADDITIONAL ACTIVITIES
- ○ Brisk Walk
- ○ Recreational Activity
- _____
- ○ Took the Stairs
- ○ Yard Work
- ○ While Watching TV
- _____
- ○ Furthest Parking Spot
- ○ Other
- _____

HOW DO I FEEL?
- ○ Totally Awesome
- ○ Energetic
- ○ Motivated
- ○ Satisfied
- ○ Hungry
- ○ Moody
- ○ Lethargic
- ○ Stressed
- ○ Need Sleep
- ○ Other
- _____

NOTES
_____
_____
_____
_____

18 DAY

M T W T F S S

BREAKFAST
- ○ Skipped It
- ○ Coffee or Tea Only
- ○ Protein 20-40g
- ○ Post Workout Carbs
- ○ Vegetables
- ○ Fat

LUNCH
- ○ Protein 20-40g
- ○ Vegetables
- ○ Fat
- ○ Post Workout Carbs

AFTERNOON SNACK
- ○ Protein 20-40g
- ○ Vegetables
- ○ Fat
- ○ Fruit

DINNER
- ○ Protein 20-40g
- ○ Vegetables
- ○ Carb Serving
- ○ Fat
- ○ Dessert

EXERCISE
- ○ Strength Training
- ○ Cardio
- _____
- ○ Other
- _____

ADDITIONAL ACTIVITIES
- ○ Brisk Walk
- ○ Recreational Activity
- _____
- ○ Took the Stairs
- ○ Yard Work
- ○ While Watching TV
- _____
- ○ Furthest Parking Spot
- ○ Other
- _____

HOW DO I FEEL?
- ○ Totally Awesome
- ○ Energetic
- ○ Motivated
- ○ Satisfied
- ○ Hungry
- ○ Moody
- ○ Lethargic
- ○ Stressed
- ○ Need Sleep
- ○ Other
- _____

NOTES
_____
_____
_____
_____

19 DAY

M T W T F S S

BREAKFAST
- ○ Skipped It
- ○ Coffee or Tea Only
- ○ Protein 20-40g
- ○ Post Workout Carbs
- ○ Vegetables
- ○ Fat

LUNCH
- ○ Protein 20-40g
- ○ Vegetables
- ○ Fat
- ○ Post Workout Carbs

AFTERNOON SNACK
- ○ Protein 20-40g
- ○ Vegetables
- ○ Fat
- ○ Fruit

DINNER
- ○ Protein 20-40g
- ○ Vegetables
- ○ Carb Serving
- ○ Fat
- ○ Dessert

EXERCISE
- ○ Strength Training
- ○ Cardio
- _____
- ○ Other
- _____

ADDITIONAL ACTIVITIES
- ○ Brisk Walk
- ○ Recreational Activity
- _____
- ○ Took the Stairs
- ○ Yard Work
- ○ While Watching TV
- _____
- ○ Furthest Parking Spot
- ○ Other
- _____

HOW DO I FEEL?
- ○ Totally Awesome
- ○ Energetic
- ○ Motivated
- ○ Satisfied
- ○ Hungry
- ○ Moody
- ○ Lethargic
- ○ Stressed
- ○ Need Sleep
- ○ Other
- _____

NOTES
_____
_____
_____
_____

20 DAY

M T W T F S S

BREAKFAST
- ○ Skipped It
- ○ Coffee or Tea Only
- ○ Protein 20-40g
- ○ Post Workout Carbs
- ○ Vegetables
- ○ Fat

LUNCH
- ○ Protein 20-40g
- ○ Vegetables
- ○ Fat
- ○ Post Workout Carbs

AFTERNOON SNACK
- ○ Protein 20-40g
- ○ Vegetables
- ○ Fat
- ○ Fruit

DINNER
- ○ Protein 20-40g
- ○ Vegetables
- ○ Carb Serving
- ○ Fat
- ○ Dessert

EXERCISE
- ○ Strength Training
- ○ Cardio
- ○ Other _____

ADDITIONAL ACTIVITIES
- ○ Brisk Walk
- ○ Recreational Activity

_____
- ○ Took the Stairs
- ○ Yard Work
- ○ While Watching TV

_____
- ○ Furthest Parking Spot
- ○ Other

_____

HOW DO I FEEL?
- ○ Totally Awesome
- ○ Energetic
- ○ Motivated
- ○ Satisfied
- ○ Hungry
- ○ Moody
- ○ Lethargic
- ○ Stressed
- ○ Need Sleep
- ○ Other

_____

NOTES
_____
_____
_____
_____

21 DAY

M T W T F S S

BREAKFAST
- ○ Skipped It
- ○ Coffee or Tea Only
- ○ Protein 20-40g
- ○ Post Workout Carbs
- ○ Vegetables
- ○ Fat

LUNCH
- ○ Protein 20-40g
- ○ Vegetables
- ○ Fat
- ○ Post Workout Carbs

AFTERNOON SNACK
- ○ Protein 20-40g
- ○ Vegetables
- ○ Fat
- ○ Fruit

DINNER
- ○ Protein 20-40g
- ○ Vegetables
- ○ Carb Serving
- ○ Fat
- ○ Dessert

EXERCISE
- ○ Strength Training
- ○ Cardio
- ○ Other _____

ADDITIONAL ACTIVITIES
- ○ Brisk Walk
- ○ Recreational Activity

_____

- ○ Took the Stairs
- ○ Yard Work
- ○ While Watching TV

_____

- ○ Furthest Parking Spot
- ○ Other

_____

HOW DO I FEEL?
- ○ Totally Awesome
- ○ Energetic
- ○ Motivated
- ○ Satisfied
- ○ Hungry
- ○ Moody
- ○ Lethargic
- ○ Stressed
- ○ Need Sleep
- ○ Other

_____

NOTES

_____
_____
_____
_____

22 DAY

M T W T F S S

BREAKFAST
- ○ Skipped It
- ○ Coffee or Tea Only
- ○ Protein 20-40g
- ○ Post Workout Carbs
- ○ Vegetables
- ○ Fat

LUNCH
- ○ Protein 20-40g
- ○ Vegetables
- ○ Fat
- ○ Post Workout Carbs

AFTERNOON SNACK
- ○ Protein 20-40g
- ○ Vegetables
- ○ Fat
- ○ Fruit

DINNER
- ○ Protein 20-40g
- ○ Vegetables
- ○ Carb Serving
- ○ Fat
- ○ Dessert

EXERCISE
- ○ Strength Training
- ○ Cardio
  _____
- ○ Other
  _____

ADDITIONAL ACTIVITIES
- ○ Brisk Walk
- ○ Recreational Activity
  _____
- ○ Took the Stairs
- ○ Yard Work
- ○ While Watching TV
  _____
- ○ Furthest Parking Spot
- ○ Other
  _____

HOW DO I FEEL?
- ○ Totally Awesome
- ○ Energetic
- ○ Motivated
- ○ Satisfied
- ○ Hungry
- ○ Moody
- ○ Lethargic
- ○ Stressed
- ○ Need Sleep
- ○ Other
  _____

NOTES
_____
_____
_____
_____

23 DAY

M T W T F S S

BREAKFAST
- ○ Skipped It
- ○ Coffee or Tea Only
- ○ Protein 20-40g
- ○ Post Workout Carbs
- ○ Vegetables
- ○ Fat

LUNCH
- ○ Protein 20-40g
- ○ Vegetables
- ○ Fat
- ○ Post Workout Carbs

AFTERNOON SNACK
- ○ Protein 20-40g
- ○ Vegetables
- ○ Fat
- ○ Fruit

DINNER
- ○ Protein 20-40g
- ○ Vegetables
- ○ Carb Serving
- ○ Fat
- ○ Dessert

EXERCISE
- ○ Strength Training
- ○ Cardio
- ○ Other _____

ADDITIONAL ACTIVITIES
- ○ Brisk Walk
- ○ Recreational Activity
- _____
- ○ Took the Stairs
- ○ Yard Work
- ○ While Watching TV
- _____
- ○ Furthest Parking Spot
- ○ Other
- _____

HOW DO I FEEL?
- ○ Totally Awesome
- ○ Energetic
- ○ Motivated
- ○ Satisfied
- ○ Hungry
- ○ Moody
- ○ Lethargic
- ○ Stressed
- ○ Need Sleep
- ○ Other
- _____

NOTES
_____
_____
_____
_____

24 DAY

M T W T F S S

BREAKFAST
- ○ Skipped It
- ○ Coffee or Tea Only
- ○ Protein 20-40g
- ○ Post Workout Carbs
- ○ Vegetables
- ○ Fat

LUNCH
- ○ Protein 20-40g
- ○ Vegetables
- ○ Fat
- ○ Post Workout Carbs

NOTES
_____
_____
_____
_____

AFTERNOON SNACK
- ○ Protein 20-40g
- ○ Vegetables
- ○ Fat
- ○ Fruit

DINNER
- ○ Protein 20-40g
- ○ Vegetables
- ○ Carb Serving
- ○ Fat
- ○ Dessert

EXERCISE
- ○ Strength Training
- ○ Cardio
- _____
- ○ Other
- _____

ADDITIONAL ACTIVITIES
- ○ Brisk Walk
- ○ Recreational Activity
- _____
- ○ Took the Stairs
- ○ Yard Work
- ○ While Watching TV
- _____
- ○ Furthest Parking Spot
- ○ Other
- _____

HOW DO I FEEL?
- ○ Totally Awesome
- ○ Energetic
- ○ Motivated
- ○ Satisfied
- ○ Hungry
- ○ Moody
- ○ Lethargic
- ○ Stressed
- ○ Need Sleep
- ○ Other
- _____

25
DAY

M T W T F S S

BREAKFAST
- ○ Skipped It
- ○ Coffee or Tea Only
- ○ Protein 20-40g
- ○ Post Workout Carbs
- ○ Vegetables
- ○ Fat

LUNCH
- ○ Protein 20-40g
- ○ Vegetables
- ○ Fat
- ○ Post Workout Carbs

AFTERNOON SNACK
- ○ Protein 20-40g
- ○ Vegetables
- ○ Fat
- ○ Fruit

DINNER
- ○ Protein 20-40g
- ○ Vegetables
- ○ Carb Serving
- ○ Fat
- ○ Dessert

EXERCISE
- ○ Strength Training
- ○ Cardio
- ○ Other _____

ADDITIONAL ACTIVITIES
- ○ Brisk Walk
- ○ Recreational Activity _____
- ○ Took the Stairs
- ○ Yard Work
- ○ While Watching TV _____
- ○ Furthest Parking Spot
- ○ Other _____

HOW DO I FEEL?
- ○ Totally Awesome
- ○ Energetic
- ○ Motivated
- ○ Satisfied
- ○ Hungry
- ○ Moody
- ○ Lethargic
- ○ Stressed
- ○ Need Sleep
- ○ Other _____

NOTES
_____
_____
_____
_____

26 DAY

M T W T F S S

BREAKFAST
- ○ Skipped It
- ○ Coffee or Tea Only
- ○ Protein 20-40g
- ○ Post Workout Carbs
- ○ Vegetables
- ○ Fat

LUNCH
- ○ Protein 20-40g
- ○ Vegetables
- ○ Fat
- ○ Post Workout Carbs

AFTERNOON SNACK
- ○ Protein 20-40g
- ○ Vegetables
- ○ Fat
- ○ Fruit

DINNER
- ○ Protein 20-40g
- ○ Vegetables
- ○ Carb Serving
- ○ Fat
- ○ Dessert

EXERCISE
- ○ Strength Training
- ○ Cardio
- ○ Other _____

ADDITIONAL ACTIVITIES
- ○ Brisk Walk
- ○ Recreational Activity

_____

- ○ Took the Stairs
- ○ Yard Work
- ○ While Watching TV

_____

- ○ Furthest Parking Spot
- ○ Other

_____

HOW DO I FEEL?
- ○ Totally Awesome
- ○ Energetic
- ○ Motivated
- ○ Satisfied
- ○ Hungry
- ○ Moody
- ○ Lethargic
- ○ Stressed
- ○ Need Sleep
- ○ Other

_____

NOTES
_____
_____
_____
_____

27 DAY

M T W T F S S

BREAKFAST
- ○ Skipped It
- ○ Coffee or Tea Only
- ○ Protein 20-40g
- ○ Post Workout Carbs
- ○ Vegetables
- ○ Fat

LUNCH
- ○ Protein 20-40g
- ○ Vegetables
- ○ Fat
- ○ Post Workout Carbs

AFTERNOON SNACK
- ○ Protein 20-40g
- ○ Vegetables
- ○ Fat
- ○ Fruit

DINNER
- ○ Protein 20-40g
- ○ Vegetables
- ○ Carb Serving
- ○ Fat
- ○ Dessert

EXERCISE
- ○ Strength Training
- ○ Cardio
- _____
- ○ Other
- _____

ADDITIONAL ACTIVITIES
- ○ Brisk Walk
- ○ Recreational Activity
- _____
- ○ Took the Stairs
- ○ Yard Work
- ○ While Watching TV
- _____
- ○ Furthest Parking Spot
- ○ Other
- _____

HOW DO I FEEL?
- ○ Totally Awesome
- ○ Energetic
- ○ Motivated
- ○ Satisfied
- ○ Hungry
- ○ Moody
- ○ Lethargic
- ○ Stressed
- ○ Need Sleep
- ○ Other
- _____

NOTES
_____
_____
_____
_____

28 DAY

M T W T F S S

BREAKFAST
- ○ Skipped It
- ○ Coffee or Tea Only
- ○ Protein 20-40g
- ○ Post Workout Carbs
- ○ Vegetables
- ○ Fat

LUNCH
- ○ Protein 20-40g
- ○ Vegetables
- ○ Fat
- ○ Post Workout Carbs

NOTES

_____
_____
_____
_____

AFTERNOON SNACK
- ○ Protein 20-40g
- ○ Vegetables
- ○ Fat
- ○ Fruit

DINNER
- ○ Protein 20-40g
- ○ Vegetables
- ○ Carb Serving
- ○ Fat
- ○ Dessert

EXERCISE
- ○ Strength Training
- ○ Cardio
- _____
- ○ Other
- _____

ADDITIONAL ACTIVITIES
- ○ Brisk Walk
- ○ Recreational Activity
- _____
- ○ Took the Stairs
- ○ Yard Work
- ○ While Watching TV
- _____
- ○ Furthest Parking Spot
- ○ Other
- _____

HOW DO I FEEL?
- ○ Totally Awesome
- ○ Energetic
- ○ Motivated
- ○ Satisfied
- ○ Hungry
- ○ Moody
- ○ Lethargic
- ○ Stressed
- ○ Need Sleep
- ○ Other
- _____

29
DAY

M T W T F S S

BREAKFAST
- ○ Skipped It
- ○ Coffee or Tea Only
- ○ Protein 20-40g
- ○ Post Workout Carbs
- ○ Vegetables
- ○ Fat

LUNCH
- ○ Protein 20-40g
- ○ Vegetables
- ○ Fat
- ○ Post Workout Carbs

AFTERNOON SNACK
- ○ Protein 20-40g
- ○ Vegetables
- ○ Fat
- ○ Fruit

DINNER
- ○ Protein 20-40g
- ○ Vegetables
- ○ Carb Serving
- ○ Fat
- ○ Dessert

EXERCISE
- ○ Strength Training
- ○ Cardio
- _____
- ○ Other
- _____

ADDITIONAL ACTIVITIES
- ○ Brisk Walk
- ○ Recreational Activity
- _____
- ○ Took the Stairs
- ○ Yard Work
- ○ While Watching TV
- _____
- ○ Furthest Parking Spot
- ○ Other
- _____

HOW DO I FEEL?
- ○ Totally Awesome
- ○ Energetic
- ○ Motivated
- ○ Satisfied
- ○ Hungry
- ○ Moody
- ○ Lethargic
- ○ Stressed
- ○ Need Sleep
- ○ Other
- _____

NOTES
_____
_____
_____
_____

30 DAY

M T W T F S S

BREAKFAST
- ○ Skipped It
- ○ Coffee or Tea Only
- ○ Protein 20-40g
- ○ Post Workout Carbs
- ○ Vegetables
- ○ Fat

LUNCH
- ○ Protein 20-40g
- ○ Vegetables
- ○ Fat
- ○ Post Workout Carbs

NOTES
_____
_____
_____
_____

AFTERNOON SNACK
- ○ Protein 20-40g
- ○ Vegetables
- ○ Fat
- ○ Fruit

DINNER
- ○ Protein 20-40g
- ○ Vegetables
- ○ Carb Serving
- ○ Fat
- ○ Dessert

EXERCISE
- ○ Strength Training
- ○ Cardio
- _____
- ○ Other
- _____

ADDITIONAL ACTIVITIES
- ○ Brisk Walk
- ○ Recreational Activity
- _____
- ○ Took the Stairs
- ○ Yard Work
- ○ While Watching TV
- _____
- ○ Furthest Parking Spot
- ○ Other
- _____

HOW DO I FEEL?
- ○ Totally Awesome
- ○ Energetic
- ○ Motivated
- ○ Satisfied
- ○ Hungry
- ○ Moody
- ○ Lethargic
- ○ Stressed
- ○ Need Sleep
- ○ Other
- _____

31 DAY

M T W T F S S

BREAKFAST
- ○ Skipped It
- ○ Coffee or Tea Only
- ○ Protein 20-40g
- ○ Post Workout Carbs
- ○ Vegetables
- ○ Fat

LUNCH
- ○ Protein 20-40g
- ○ Vegetables
- ○ Fat
- ○ Post Workout Carbs

NOTES
_____
_____
_____
_____

AFTERNOON SNACK
- ○ Protein 20-40g
- ○ Vegetables
- ○ Fat
- ○ Fruit

DINNER
- ○ Protein 20-40g
- ○ Vegetables
- ○ Carb Serving
- ○ Fat
- ○ Dessert

EXERCISE
- ○ Strength Training
- ○ Cardio
  _____
- ○ Other
  _____

ADDITIONAL ACTIVITIES
- ○ Brisk Walk
- ○ Recreational Activity

  _____
- ○ Took the Stairs
- ○ Yard Work
- ○ While Watching TV

  _____
- ○ Furthest Parking Spot
- ○ Other

  _____

HOW DO I FEEL?
- ○ Totally Awesome
- ○ Energetic
- ○ Motivated
- ○ Satisfied
- ○ Hungry
- ○ Moody
- ○ Lethargic
- ○ Stressed
- ○ Need Sleep
- ○ Other

  _____

Made in the USA
Lexington, KY
25 March 2019